Essential Skills for Influencing in Healthcare

D0892533

A guide on how to influence others with integrity and success

ANDREW PRICE

Leadership Development Consultant, Bristol

and

ANDREW SCOWCROFT

Managing Director
Development Consultancy, Llantrisant

Radcliffe Publishing
London • New York

Radcliffe Publishing Ltd
33–41 Dallington Street
London
EC1V 0BB
United Kingdom

www.radcliffepublishing.com

British Library Cataloguing in Publication Data

A catalogue record for this book is available from the British Library.

ISBN-13: 978 184619 538 9

The paper used for the text pages of this book
is FSC® certified. FSC (The Forest Stewardship
Council®) is an international network to promote
responsible management of the world's forests.

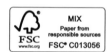

Typeset by Phoenix Photosetting, Chatham, Kent
Printed and bound by TJI Digital, Padstow, Cornwall

Contents

Preface

THE PURPOSE OF THIS BOOK

The purpose of this book is to improve the practice of influencing others, as carried out by managers and clinicians in healthcare environments. We believe that those roles have a vital part to play in motivating, inspiring and influencing their staff to do the best they can in the workplace. However, our observations and experiences of influencing behaviours are that they often produce low-level commitment, flawed or unsustainable change outcomes and, ironically, staff who are even less inclined to be influenced next time.

There is no shortage of issues to be addressed in healthcare, and no shortage of good ideas. What is often lacking is an approach to influencing change that has genuine integrity and trust built in from the start. And integrity is not just a word or a vaguely held value. It has to be demonstrated practically through the way managers and clinicians engage with their colleagues.

For you the reader, our hope is that this book will help you:

➤ be more optimistic and hopeful about people at work
➤ recognise your potential to bring about positive change
➤ understand yourself and your impact on others better
➤ feel that the management part of your job is a high calling
➤ have confidence to listen to and trust your staff
➤ take practical steps to bring about a change in your practice.

Andrew Price and Andrew Scowcroft
September 2011

About the authors

ANDREW PRICE MSC, MHSM, DIPHSM

Andrew's main focus is on leadership and team development, helping people to work positively and effectively with each other. He works as a freelance consultant in the public, private and voluntary sectors.

Andrew moved into consultancy after a career in NHS management. During this time he moved from hospital management into leadership development, and his final NHS role was as the acting chief executive of the Centre for Health Leadership.

Andrew has an MSc in Leadership and Organisation in the Public Sector from the University of the West of England. He also has a Diploma in Health Management and is a member of the Institute of Health Management. He has published in a number of journals including *Health Service Journal*, *Health Management* and *Public Policy Review*. Between 2008 and 2011 he was the Chair of One25, an award-winning charity working with abused and disadvantaged women

Andrew lives in Bristol and is married to Ruth, a dance movement psychotherapist. They have two daughters.

ANDREW SCOWCROFT MA, MHSM, MCIPD, FINST LM

Andrew is an experienced and respected management development consultant and health service manager, with 37 years' public sector experience, including 20 years as a self-financing consultant.

He is frequently engaged by the NHS and other public and private sector clients to provide a range of services, from training and development programmes through to executive coaching for top managers. Andrew has a strong commitment to releasing the potential of leaders and managers, and their organisations, and his development activities are extremely highly rated due to the practical nature of the material and its rapid transferability to the workplace.

With Andrew Price, he has developed Vital Signs, a suite of foundational management skills programmes for managers, and has received endorsement from the Institute of Leadership and Management for these courses.

Andrew has a Diploma from the Institute of Health Services Management, BPS Level A and B certificates in Psychometric Testing, and an MA in Learning and Change in Organisations, from the University of the West of England.

Andrew lives in Llantrisant, South Wales, is married to Ann, an occupational therapist, and they have two daughters.

Both Andrews can be contacted via www.developmentconsultancy.co.uk.

Acknowledgements

Many people have inspired, enabled and contributed to the writing of this book. Much of the book is drawn from our Vital Signs 2 programme and we are grateful to those clients who decided to invest in training that looked a little different from most others. Ann Price, Virginia Spight and Kim Tovey, take a bow! We love running this programme, principally because of the energy, honesty and intellect of the healthcare staff we work with. Many of the case studies in the book come from Vital Signs participants and we're grateful to them for sharing their stories with us. Thanks especially to Rachel Armitage for letting us quote from her assignment.

We'd also like to thank Gillian Nineham at Radcliffe for her encouragement in getting the book finished and Ashleigh Dunn, Steffi Williams and, again, Kim Tovey for taking the time to plough through the manuscript and offer their thoughts. Nicola Hartnell not only provided much needed office support but also revealed a considerable talent for drawing cartoons.

Others have been responsible for inspiring in us the thought that we had something worth writing. Not least among these was our former boss, the late Professor Stephen Prosser, whose words and example and friendship were so influential.

Above all, though, we are thankful for our families who have been so supportive and patient. Ann, Claire and Hannah, Ruth, Abbie and Roanna, you are a source of joy.

Dedicated to Ann and Ruth
(*Proverbs* 18:22)

Introduction

To influence someone is to bring about some modification in their beliefs, attitudes or behaviour through your behaviour towards them. Of the many ways to do this, here are five significant and common approaches.

➤ The *first* is to use force. Through fear, your own formidable physical presence or by overwhelming the other party with sheer numbers of allies, you can try to force through the change you want to see.

➤ The *second* is by laws and rules. This includes not only the legal framework of national laws but also the rules inside organisations that impose structures and procedures. These in turn create the power of hierarchical authority that can impose change. Another version of this is the power of reward and sanction – having the right to grant or withhold permission – again often associated with seniority and job status.

There are a couple of serious flaws in these first two approaches. The first, and the principal reason why this book has been written, is that it is too easy for integrity to be sacrificed in the blind pursuit of compliance from others. When the pressure is on, an organisation's fixation on performance and targets can lead to a mindset that believes ends will always justify means, and a tacit corporate endorsement of any collateral damage amongst the staff. The second flaw is that the resultant changes are rarely sustainable. They rely on the continuation of force or authority to keep the compliance in place.

➤ The *third* approach uses technical expertise. If you are an acknowledged expert on a particular topic then it is relatively easy to use that fact to bring about change in others. Note, the expertise itself is normally neutral. It is the intentions of the expert that will determine whether the knowledge will be a force for good or for harm.

➤ The *fourth* is by manipulation, either intellectual or psychological. Most of us know of colleagues who are good with words or just have a knack of getting their own way and you are left wondering afterwards – how did they get me to do that?

1

This fourth approach appears quite attractive, particularly if we are the ones doing the clever word play, but there is still a problem. Whilst the approach will work, it will only work once! The next time, the victim will remember being outmanoeuvred, be far more wary and suspicious, and, as a consequence, far harder to persuade – regardless of the merits of the current argument. Over time, these 'manipulators' acquire a reputation that actually reduces rather than enhances their influencing ability. In other words, it is possible to be too clever for your own good.

➤ The *fifth* and final approach is influencing with integrity, an approach that requires a genuine attempt to understand and then work with the personality, views and concerns of the other person, seeking to involve them in co-designing the desired change and so produce sustainable outcomes. This is the approach we explore in this book.

If you are the type of manager who enjoys exerting your authority, intimidating your colleagues or using your unique expertise to win intellectual battles, you probably still need this book but will need courage and an open mind to read any further.

However, if you want to place integrity at the centre of your management practice, then you will find this book invaluable.

Most of us would admit that, when other people want us to do something, we would appreciate being treated with respect and that, if we have any reservations about the request, we would like these listened to and taken into account. In other words, if we do not want to go along with the plan, we are not being difficult, we are simply the voice of reason and good sense!

However, when we are the one doing the requesting, speed is of the essence, our bosses expect results, and we haven't got time to consult with everyone. Those who object or get in the way are quickly labelled as resistors, to be forced or sidelined!

This unintentional hypocrisy lies behind many of the struggles faced by organisations and their staff as they grapple with change. Time after time, frontline staff and local managers report that they are simply not treated genuinely by their corporate bosses, and time after time Boards and senior managers are frustrated at the slow pace of change lower down the organisation.

A multinational IBM survey in 2008[1] revealed that an average of nearly 60% of all organisational change projects fail to achieve some or all of their objectives, and in some cases the figure was as high as 80%. Given the arguments we have already put forward, it is unsurprising to read the IBM researcher's conclusion that one of the main reasons for this poor success rate was the difficulty in changing mindsets. And if organisations continue to treat the influencing process as simply the task of issuing new edicts and demanding compliance, via the issuing of group emails (what we call 'sheep dipping'), then those sad statistics are likely to continue for some time.

In this book we will not only argue that integrity and ethical influencing work, we will give you the insights and techniques to make it a reality. Of course, there may still be times when the circumstances call for a quick dose of orders and obedience, but we believe your staff will be more ready to accept those if they too see the genuine need for speed on this occasion, and they feel involved, respected and trusted the rest of the time.

If there is one central belief that runs through this whole book, it is that people, if treated well, are worthy of immense trust. Think for a moment. When away from the workplace, your staff spend their whole lives doing amazing and complex things, such as bringing up a family, organising their finances, arranging holidays, navigating traffic, supporting elderly relatives, running charities, building houses, handling bereavement and executing wills, and operating second businesses. Who gave them a manual for all of that? Who checked their time sheets? Who told them how to work together to achieve these things? No one. They thought it through for themselves and then got on and made things happen. Yes, they made mistakes, and used those experiences to make next time better.

Now consider the degree of self-determination and freedom to innovate that those same people have in your workplace. For some, the comparison will be a positive one. For many, though, it will reveal that your people are capable of more, much more. But, and it is a significant but, only if they are managed, influenced and supported, ethically and with integrity in the workplace.

As you work your way through this book, we invite you to pause at intervals and bring to the front of your mind situations that might benefit from the approaches offered. Unless you combine your real-world experiences with the advice we offer, there is little chance of the book achieving its purpose.

There are six main chapters to this book, each covering one theme or topic, followed by a summary chapter.

CHAPTER 1: LEARNING TO INFLUENCE

This chapter analyses the factors that can stop you and your team from learning from your unsuccessful influencing experiences and suggests how you can remove those blockages.

CHAPTER 2: LEARNING ABOUT YOURSELF

This chapter looks at you, how you tend to go about influencing others, where that might work and where it can go wrong. By raising your awareness of your own preferences, you will be better able to identify the (often different) preferences of others and so modify your approaches accordingly.

CHAPTER 3: ORGANISATIONAL CULTURE

Here we explore the different routines, rituals and (unwritten) rules that exist inside teams, departments and whole organisations. These are often described as the culture of that organisation and if you can successfully diagnose the prevailing culture of the people you are trying to influence, you can then fine-tune your approach to meet their needs.

CHAPTER 4: INFLUENCING ORGANISATIONAL CHANGE

The foundations of our thinking about change lie in an approach to management that is more mechanical than human. This leads to change by force which is unsustainable and leaves people bruised. In this chapter we suggest how change can be influenced in a way that recognises that organisations are made up of people.

CHAPTER 5: INFLUENCING IN FORMAL SETTINGS

Whilst much of your influencing will take place in informal settings, during other meetings, and even away from the workplace at times, there will be occasions where the parties need to convene in a room and do some face-to-face bargaining. This chapter will offer advice on how to both manage the overall process and conduct your own part in the negotiations with professionalism and dignity.

CHAPTER 6: BEING A ROLE MODEL

This chapter looks at how you manage yourself. This is important because, in the eyes of those around you (staff, peers, bosses, etc.), how you cope in the job will either add to or detract from your personal credibility and influence.

CHAPTER 7: SUMMARY AND NEXT STEPS

This final chapter summarises the main messages from the previous chapters and helps you to decide what you can do to put some of the lessons of the book into action.

Two caveats …

In writing a book about integrity and ethics, it is only fair that the book represents itself accurately. Therefore, before you read any further, there are two important things to say about what the book is not!

First, it is not a book about how to come up with good ideas and proposals to take to other people. There are plenty of worthy publications covering that topic. What we will say is that if your case is a poor one then no amount of influencing (ethical or otherwise) will improve its chances. To quote the old saying, 'you cannot make a silk purse out of a sow's ear'.

Second, the book is not part of the 'three easy steps to ...' family of management guides. Our difficulty with such checklist publications is that, despite their brevity and ease of reading, you will never really know what is behind a particular technique and why it did or did not work if all you have to go on is a list of one-liner bullet points. This book avoids theory for theory's sake but does invite you to dig a little deeper and learn why different approaches work as they do. That way, you will be better able to adapt the advice to fit your circumstances rather than trying to fit your circumstances to a rather rigid set of prescribed bullet points.

Having cleared our authors' consciences, we invite you now to read on. We truly hope you find ways of enhancing the integrity of your influencing practice.

REFERENCE

1 IBM Corporation. *Making Change Work*. Somers, NY: IBM Corporation; 2008. www-935.ibm.com/services/us/gbs/bus/html/gbs-making-change-work.html

CHAPTER 1

Learning to influence

Personally I'm always ready to learn, although I do not always like being taught.

(Winston Churchill)

This book could profoundly alter the way you influence people, or it could leave you unchanged. The difference will lie in the extent to which you are ready to learn. And by 'learn' we don't mean acquire facts. The sort of learning we need to do to become effective in influencing encompasses values, attitudes and behaviour, not just information. So we will start with the issue of learning.

This chapter focuses on the things that can prevent you learning to become a more effective influencer and how you can overcome them. We're not talking about external factors here, but internal ones such as our assumptions about people and the way things should be done which can either prevent or enable learning. These internal factors matter more than IQ when it comes to real learning, by which we mean learning that changes us. More than just cleverness is required to change the way we deal with people; humility is also needed. Unless we are prepared to change, why should those around us do so?

LEARNING DOESN'T HAPPEN AUTOMATICALLY

Much of what we have written in this book is already in the public domain. We do not lay claim to any trade secrets or fresh revelations. And quite apart from what can be found in books, each day of our lives brings new opportunities to learn and change. For us, the really interesting question is that with all this knowledge available so widely, and with daily experience as a rich potential source of learning, how come individuals, teams and organisations seem to find it so hard to learn to change what they do?

Imagine if learning automatically took place every time we were exposed to a learning opportunity, and we always accepted the lessons that experience offered. Our organisations would be very different. We would all become steadily wiser and more effective throughout our working lives and pass on this learning to younger colleagues who would be keen to listen. Our work would be progressively improving in all aspects as learning is passed on. We would never make the same mistake twice and innovative practice would be quickly adopted. The reality is often very different. Organisations and people within them often seem to find learning, and the changes that go with it, difficult. This is reflected in the fact that organisational learning has been a major theme in management literature since the 1990s and interest in the subject shows no sign of waning.

Changing how people work is notoriously difficult and, more often than not, it fails.[1] In a field as vital as healthcare, an expert group chaired by the Chief Medical Officer for England admitted: 'The NHS has no reliable way of identifying serious lapses ... analysing them systematically, learning from them and introducing change which sticks so as to prevent similar events from reoccurring'.[2] And, as we all know, doing something for a long time may or may not lead to improved performance. Twenty years' experience may mean the steady accumulation of a wealth of wisdom or it may mean one year's experience, repeated 19 times. We can only conclude that there is more to learning than simply being exposed to opportunities to learn. Other factors must be involved which can obstruct or enhance learning. This chapter invites you to recognise the things that stop you learning and overcome them.

THE CHALLENGE OF REAL LEARNING

Some learning is simple. You may learn that a certain combination of keys on your computer keyboard is a shortcut, saving you precious time with a regular task. You already knew how to use a computer and you are familiar with the idea of shortcuts, but you have now added another one to your repertoire. Or your professional studies might provide knowledge of an area that, hitherto, you knew little or nothing about. The gap is filled in and you now possess more information. You note or memorise the new data and incorporate it into your work, but it fits neatly alongside other things you already knew or builds on more basic professional knowledge you already possess.

But other learning may be more of a struggle. In his early management career, Andrew Price saw himself as an energetic, decisive but compassionate manager. He wasn't sure exactly how he had formed this view but it fitted in with his vague ideas of what good management was and the sort of person he'd like to be. When he moved from operational management in hospitals to a leadership training department, he was exposed to self-assessment tools, personality tests and to people skilled in giving feedback. Over time, he was confronted with compelling evidence from several sources that, in fact, people saw him as slightly withdrawn, sometimes slow to reach a decision and reluctant to take centre stage. At first, he resisted the picture that was emerging. Was he the decisive, heart-on-his-sleeve powerhouse he had imagined or this more thoughtful, introverted type who often left decisions for as long as he could? But although he struggled with the feedback because it did not fit with the way he had seen himself, he had to admit that it did explain a lot. He began to realise why he had not enjoyed certain roles, particularly those which allowed little time for reflection and involved almost constant activity. The part he struggled with most was the realisation that although he genuinely felt compassionate and concerned for the people he managed, he did not often display it. All of this led to a succession of changes, from a conscious decision to be more openly encouraging and supportive, to a resetting of career goals. Learning had taken place, but it had been neither quick nor easy. At the heart of Andrew's struggle was the tension between the feedback he was receiving from other people and the idea he had of himself.

A more dramatic example from popular culture is the 1996 film *Jerry Maguire* which starred Tom Cruise. The hero is a sports agent who, after suffering a nervous breakdown, realises his career and much of his industry are based on deceit and dishonesty. This realisation, this new learning, leads him to make significant changes in his behaviour and he decides to work with uncompromising integrity from then on. The film shows the cost of this learning as clients and friends are mystified or even alienated by his transformation. What he learns about himself leads to profound changes in how he conducts his relationships and how he does business.

TWO TYPES OF LEARNING

The difference between the first examples and the later ones is that for Andrew, and for the character in the film, the learning could not just be slotted in alongside what they already knew. Instead, it challenged what they had previously believed and how they had previously acted. This was disruptive learning: learning that displaced rather than augmented. The challenge for Andrew was to let go of how he saw himself and accept a more realistic, and ultimately more helpful, self-image. This required time and painful honesty. Learning a computer shortcut or filling in the gaps in your technical knowledge tend to present much less of a challenge.

These two types of learning correspond to some extent with Piaget's idea of learning by assimilation and learning by accommodation.[3] The former is where the learner can easily perceive, understand and act on the new information. The latter, however, requires 'an internal structural change in your beliefs, ideas and attitudes',[4] something easier said than done. When we talk about learning to influence, the learning required is mainly learning by accommodation. When we run our Vital Signs management development programmes, we make the point that the only learning that matters is learning that results in changed behaviour. Giving people more theories or facts about management will not, in itself, change behaviour. And without a change in our behaviour – what we do, how we communicate and how we deal with people – there is no change in our managing or influencing.

METANOIA: CHANGING YOUR MIND

In English, we use the term 'learning' for both the acquisition of knowledge which may be trivial and for profound alterations in how we think and act. Peter Senge[5] makes the point that a better word exists for profound learning but it has fallen out of use. *Metanoia* is a Greek word meaning a change of mind or a change in our thinking. In ancient religious tradition, it signifies a fundamental transformation or mind-shift. It conveys the idea that to make significant changes in how we behave, significant changes in our thinking are required.

This deeper, more disruptive learning is necessary if we are to become effective influencers. For this reason, we encourage you to expect some degree of struggle as you put your knowledge into practice. Indeed, it is in the areas where you encounter the greatest difficulty that the potential for learning may be greatest as your deeply held assumptions and values are challenged. But without this willingness to struggle, to work with the concepts in practice, it remains an academic exercise.

DEFENDING AGAINST LEARNING

It is this struggle that leads us to avoid learning. We are aware that this sounds heretical but, as individuals and organisations, we have many ingenious ways of avoiding any learning that challenges existing ways of thinking or acting. It is this that explains why it is not enough simply for there to be opportunities to learn. Such opportunities may be ignored, spurned or not even recognised. When we talk about these defences against learning on our programmes, a common response is for people to say 'My boss should be on this course'. It is much easier to see where other people, particularly those whose seniority means they are more exposed to scrutiny, are going wrong. In fact, as we will see, a readiness to criticise others can in itself be a way of avoiding personal learning. But you will gain much more from this chapter if you use it to reflect on your own willingness to learn and change.

Defence 1: 'It's their fault!'

We've taken the name of this defence from a remark made by a client some years ago. One of us was working with a group of nurses, whose ward had received a large number of complaints, to help them think through what action they needed to take. After a morning of reflection and analysis resulting in a wall covered in flip-chart diagrams and drawings, the ward manager gave us her conclusion. 'It's a blame culture here,' she said, '... and it's their fault!'

This defence works by finding fault with someone else and thereby absolving ourselves of the need to learn. 'It's their fault,' we point out, 'so I don't need to change'. Of course, our use of this defence, because we all employ it from time to time, is usually much more subtle.

It works like this. Perhaps you have been trying to influence your boss to support an initiative you are convinced will improve the work of your team. Your proposal is turned down and as you walk away disappointed from the meeting, there is a strong temptation to locate the reason for the setback with your boss. He is too cautious, you might think, he cannot see the real issues. You may accuse the boss, silently or in private with your friends, of plain stupidity. If this is not the first time this has happened, you console yourself in the next team meeting by saying how typical it is for him to act this way.

Blaming others is all too common. 'It's those idiots in finance/IT/headquarters' is a common response when our influencing has not led to the desired result. Of course, our criticisms may contain some truth, but that is not the point. Locating the fault elsewhere distracts us from the lessons that we can learn. Focusing on the real or imagined failings of others saves us asking ourselves difficult questions about the way *we* went about influencing them.

Or imagine you have been involved in a project run jointly with another organisation or agency. The course of action that seemed so obvious to you is causing them anxiety and they have referred the decision back to their top management, causing yet more delays. What is your response? You could storm away from the meeting, muttering the word 'bureaucrats' under your breath. If this is the course of action you choose, you will avoid the discomfort of learning but make it very likely that you will repeat the experience next time.

However, the *learning* response is to step back from the situation and see what you could do, or could have done, differently. On reflection, you see that the more you push them to agree with you, the more anxious they become. The more you disparage their way of working, which seems to you to be so bureaucratic, the more they insist on protocol. You have an uncomfortable realisation that you may have been part of the problem. You begin to see lessons which, even if it is too late for this project, can help next time.

Storming out of the meeting would only confirm for the other agency that, in view of your impulsiveness and unco-operative behaviour, they were right to be so careful. Your display of temper will, if anything, lead them to adopt an even more cautious approach in future. Whereas an appreciation of your own role in shaping their behaviour might lead to a more constructive response. It may be difficult, faced with what you see as time-wasting, to remain calm and helpful but that is more likely to keep the process moving forward. You could even ask whether there is anything you could do which would help them in their decision making.

On a residential NHS management development course some years ago, a visiting speaker arrived the night before his session and began to 'bond' with the group of trainees over dinner and the chat in the lounge afterwards. The intention was honourable but he tried too hard (joining in with the 'in-jokes' and copying the irreverent banter going on between group members), and ended up alienating some of the group. The following morning, several people decided to skip that speaker's session, explaining later that the man 'was a bit of a fool'. Perhaps so but those people missed an opportunity to learn about the man's specialist subject, because they had fallen into a self-made trap that 'people can only learn from people they like'. Instead of struggling to reconcile their character assessment with the fact that the speaker was both senior in his field *and* offered a fascinating insight into forthcoming changes in health commissioning, they took the easy way out. A learning opportunity was missed.

Even when those we are trying to influence are behaving, in our view, badly, there is little to be achieved by blaming them in private or to their faces. It may bring a moment of satisfaction as we 'get it off our chest' but we are missing the opportunity to change the one thing we can control: our own behaviour.

We can blame or we can learn, but we can't do both. The more we see the reasons for setbacks in the behaviour of others, the less time and energy we have to fix what is wrong with ourselves.

Defence 2: Something must be done!

This is where we see the need to do something to rescue or rectify the situation, and those around us are expecting us to be decisive, so we take action. But because the action does not stem from a real understanding of the issue, we just make it worse. Have you ever tried to push a door open only to find that it will not budge? More force is applied and perhaps a swift kick, and still nothing happens. Finally you put your shoulder to the door and shove. Still nothing. It's only when you have bruised your shoulder and sworn a few times that, with embarrassment, you notice the small sign saying 'pull'.

The 'something must be done!' defence works in exactly the same way. We encounter a setback and so that we can appear to be on top of the situation, we take action. But either because we do not take time to think it through or because we don't know what else to do, the action we take will not help. However, we can at least defend ourselves. We did do *something*. We see this defence frequently in organisations as, in response to the latest scandal, they set up an inquiry or call in consultants. Not that there is anything wrong, *per se*, with either of these responses. But they are often knee-jerk reactions, or attempts to be seen to be doing something, rather than a considered response to the problem. By the time the inquiry finishes or the consultants submit their report, we have all moved on and the problem sinks from view, only to re-emerge in a slightly different guise in the future.

One hospital engineer had a tricky influencing problem. To meet the objectives her boss had set for her, she had to carry out routine maintenance on several machines needed in the operating theatres. This would require the closure of each of the theatres in turn. The operating theatres manager was reluctant to allow this, as to meet *her* boss's targets she had to keep the theatres open as long as possible to allow the maximum number of operations to be performed. Stalemate.

The engineer's initial reponse, fuelled by frustration, was to consider calling in some more senior firepower and asking her boss to try and make the theatres manager comply. After all, 'something must be done!'. This would have inevitably led to the theatres manager calling in support from *her* boss and the problem escalating through the hierarchy. The issue would not have been resolved but the engineer could salve her conscience with the thought that something had been done and action had been taken. Thankfully, a wise colleague suggested a compromise to both parties which involved temporarily extending the opening hours of some theatres to cover the one out of action due to maintenance. On reflection, it was a simple and obvious solution but one which had escaped the parties involved when all they could think of was how to achieve their individual objectives. When they widened their perspective to consider the position of the other person, a way forward became possible. The 'something must be done!' approach would have, in the end, taken longer as the senior managers slugged it out and it would have also left a legacy of ill feeling.

THE CONSEQUENCES OF 'SOMETHING MUST BE DONE'

Jake Chapman[6] gives this example of action which was taken without sufficient thought. In 2001 a large sum of money was given to those ambulance services in England which most needed to improve their performance. They used the money to recruit more staff. The problem was that many of the staff recruited moved from neighbouring ambulance services which, as a direct result, suffered from higher turnover and the costs of recruiting and training replacement staff. This was an unintended consequence, but nevertheless one which could have been foreseen. When we treat complex issues as if they were simple, such unintended consequences may detract from or even wipe out the benefits of our actions.

In some parts of the UK, there was a political decision to abolish hospital car-parking charges. The decision was welcomed by patient groups and the general public, and followed a high-profile campaign which focused on the 'injustice of the sick and their relatives having to pay to come to hospital'. Within days of the implementation, many hospital car parks began to fill up with vehicles belonging to shoppers and commuters enjoying free parking, making it more difficult for staff or visitors to find a space. In addition, the fact that some hospitals had only just negotiated long-term contracts for the management of their car parks when the announcement was made meant that in some hospitals, there were no charges and in others the charges continued for several more years.

We are not making any party political points here, but this sort of 'something must be done' decision can end up creating both the opposite of what was intended *and* a new injustice. The need to be seen to be decisive and win public support for a decision can obscure issues of long-term sustainability. Furthermore, the pace of political life means there is little time to reflect and learn for next time.

If our initial attempts to influence fail, it is hard to resist the urge to just push harder: more presentations, more forceful language or more political pressure. But before we act, we need to consider why our initial attempt failed. It may be that by doing more of the same, we may make the situation worse, not better.

Defence 3: Treating the symptoms

Like the other two, this defence is an easy one for busy managers to fall into using. Because we are faced with a multitude of pressing problems, we are happy to do things which just make them go away, or seem to go away, so we have time to deal with other things. We may not take time to see that the same issues keep recurring and that we are dealing with symptoms rather than the underlying cause.

Stephen ran the leadership training college of a large organisation. Another senior manager, Alan, who was very powerful and influential in the same organisation, was a constant thorn in his side, questioning his decisions, raising concerns over value for money and generally making life difficult. For a while, Stephen's response to this was to defend each attack and to argue his case vigorously, but this only seemed to provoke more attacks. The situation was rapidly descending into the sort of departmental sniping that can persist for years and sour relationships between people who ought to work together. After a while, Stephen concluded that he was only addressing the symptoms of a larger issue. So he changed his tactics and met with his critic during a lull in hostilities. It quickly became clear that Alan had serious reservations about the effectiveness of the programmes being run at the college and felt the money could be better spent elsewhere. At this point Stephen made a brave choice. Convinced of the quality of his programmes but ready to learn, he invited Alan to lead a review of the college. Rather than fighting him off, he asked for his advice. The result of the review was that Alan became a supporter, albeit a constructively critical one, of the college and Stephen learned some useful but uncomfortable lessons from Alan's probing review. Instead of dealing with the symptoms of Alan's scepticism, Stephen faced and dealt with the underlying issue.

This defence occurs frequently in organisational life. A common example is the way we work longer and longer hours rather than learn to deal with the central issue of an unreasonable workload or the need to develop more effective ways of working. Not only do we not deal with the issue, we set up a vicious circle whereby work pressures create domestic pressures which in turn make it harder for us to perform well at work. It is all too easy to find ourselves avoiding uncomfortable learning by dealing with the symptoms.

The way to avoid merely treating the symptoms involves taking time to reflect and to listen carefully to the people involved. Later in this chapter, we'll suggest some exercises which will help with reflection and listening, but there is no quick fix. Make up your mind to become a good managerial diagnostician, able to see through to root causes.

WHY SMART PEOPLE DON'T LEARN

In his perceptive study of senior staff in an American consultancy firm, entitled 'Teaching smart people how to learn',[7] Chris Argyris unearthed two powerful reasons for the way we, without thinking, avoid lessons that could help us.

One is the desire to save face. Almost all learning involves an admission that we were previously either wrong or ignorant. Particularly for senior people, it can be hard to be humble, and face-saving can lead to all kinds of mental and moral gymnastics as we try to preserve the appearance of always being right. Put like this, it sounds both ridiculous and indefensible, but few of us are completely free of the desire to look clever.

Another reason is the lack of practice smart people have in failing. To quote Argyris, 'Because many professionals are almost always successful at what they do, they rarely experience failure. And because they have rarely failed, they have never learned how to learn from failure. So whenever their ... strategies go wrong, they become defensive, screen out criticism and put the "blame" on anyone and everyone but themselves. In short, their ability to learn shuts down at the moment they need it the most'.

CHANGING OUR MENTAL MODELS

Another thing that limits our learning is what Gary Hamel calls 'the drag of old mental models'.[8] These are beliefs which we do not question, we 'just know' that they are true. They could be beliefs about people, organisations or society in general. They may have been passed on to us from parents, teachers or influential figures in our professional life or we may just somehow have absorbed them during our lives. Their power lies in the fact that they are the givens, the unchallenged assumptions in any thought process, shaping the way we think and limiting our ability to innovate and learn.

We can smile at many of the beliefs once accepted as fact which were subsequently proved false. Large numbers of people at different times 'just knew' that:

➤ women should not be educated
➤ personality could be deduced from the size and shape of the head
➤ the sun revolves around the earth
➤ illness is caused by an imbalance in the four humours.

But if history shows anything about mental models, it is that we all possess them and they are remarkably persistent. It is very easy to identify examples of mental models that have no basis in fact but which are still widely believed, such as the idea that we only use 10% of our brains or that stomach ulcers are caused by stress or spicy food or that playing Mozart to your children will make them more intelligent.[9]

Another commonly held mental model, which we still hear on our courses, is 'people don't like change'. This can often be decoded as 'my attempts at influencing have failed, so that proves people don't like change'. As you will read in the chapter on influencing change, this 'just know' mental model is simply false.

As well as these widely held mental models, we have personal assumptions which affect how we deal with people and situations. We are often not conscious of them, and it is this invisibility which makes them so hard to recognise and deal with. In learning to influence, the danger of unchallenged mental models is that we will reject information or courses of action that conflict with what we 'just know' to be true. If I believe that staff, particularly those in low-paid manual work, will always do the minimum and cannot think for themselves, then I will always act in a way that is controlling and patronising. I will never be able to engage the initiative and creativity of my employees in the way that enabled Toyota to steal a march on its American competitors[8] or that helped Ricardo Semler turn his company, SEMCO, into a profitable experiment in workplace democracy.[10] Semler turned conventional wisdom on its head by involving staff in setting their own hours and even their own salaries. Many of his peers 'just knew' it wouldn't work, but it did and business thrived.

If I 'just know' that all medical staff are arrogant, all accountants lack imagination or that all managers are paper-pushers, I will be unable to find common ground with them and any attempt to influence them with integrity is likely to fail. Also, my prejudice may well leak out into my behaviour which, again, will make a successful outcome unlikely.

THE POWER OF ASSUMPTIONS

Douglas McGregor[11] argued that behind every managerial act or decision lies an assumption about people at work. He set out two broad categories of assumptions called theory X and theory Y.

Theory X assumptions	Theory Y assumptions
People don't like work	Work is as natural as rest or play
People need to be coerced or threatened to work	Work can be a source of satisfaction
People avoid responsibility and prefer to be told what to do	Provided they are committed to organisational goals, people will exercise self-direction and self-control
People need to be encouraged to do good work	People want to do a good job

Our assumptions about people become a self-fulfilling prophecy. If a manager's assumptions are in line with theory X, he will tend to monitor his staff closely, allowing them little freedom. This behaviour will eventually demotivate his staff, as they begin to feel they are not trusted or even that they are incompetent. Staff who feel like this are unlikely to show initiative or enjoy their work. The staff's lack of motivation and drive is seen by the manager as proof that they need even more control.

Are you theory X or theory Y?

SINGLE- AND DOUBLE-LOOP LEARNING

Chris Argyris[12] has illustrated how these unchallenged and often flawed mental models can restrict our learning. Single-loop learning is when we respond to circumstances according to our existing beliefs and assumptions. Argyris compares this to a thermostat, which is programmed to turn the heating on and off to maintain a certain temperature. It can 'learn', in that it responds to the circumstances and takes corrective action, but it can only do so within limits. The thermostat cannot alter its own settings. It cannot question whether the temperature is the right one or decide not to turn the heating on because no one is at home. If the thermostat were able to question and change its settings, this would be double-loop learning. In single-loop learning, we may refine existing practice but we cannot fundamentally challenge it. Double-loop learning entails a conscious change to the mental models that drive our behaviour.

If my approach to influencing is based on the assumption that people are only driven by either their desire for material reward or their fear of punishment, I will probably notice that I am not always successful. So I might refine my technique, looking for more attractive rewards in the shape of pay or other benefits or employing a bigger stick such as tighter controls over how people work. I could research the very latest types of bonus schemes or performance management, but I am still being driven by the same basic assumption, i.e. that staff are driven only by greed or fear. The fundamental flaw is that many people do their best work when inspired by a sense of meaning or higher purpose. The power of loyalty or the satisfaction that comes from helping vulnerable people is ignored by the mindset that sees fear and greed as the only real motivators.

Unless I become aware of my mental model, I can never address the flaw in my influencing. I can only get better and better at doing the wrong thing! The urge to make a difference is a powerful one and wise managers are acknowledging that if we give them the opportunity, staff want to be part of work that 'raises them to higher levels of motivation and morality'.[13] To accept that the search for meaning and the desire to make a positive difference to the world are powerful motivations entails a change to my mental model. This is double-loop learning.

INFLUENCING NHS STAFF

A report by the Nuffield Foundation argues that 'NHS staff are motivated by the opportunity to deliver high-quality services'.[14] While staff are also motivated by good working conditions and other factors, it is noticeable that successive NHS reforms seem to ignore this potentially dynamic motivating factor. Instead, they focus more on ensuring implementation through targets rather than tapping into the desire of NHS staff to improve care.[15] Or, put another way, reforms have tended to focus more on controlling behaviour rather than releasing potential. This is both a mistake and a missed opportunity. Our experience in working with all types of NHS staff is that most will go to great lengths to change or improve their practice *provided* they see a benefit for patients.

What makes double-loop learning so hard is that we are mostly unaware of our own mental models, our 'givens'. They lie beneath the surface until they are challenged. For many managers, a crude carrot-and-stick approach to influencing behaviour is not a belief they have arrived at through thoughtful consideration; it is not that they have consciously chosen to adopt this assumption. Like much conventional wisdom, it is just somehow absorbed as being true.

Another barrier to double-loop learning is that when we begin to question these commonly held assumptions, we are likely to encounter ridicule or resistance. Many years ago, one of us was part of a team attempting to set up the first training programme in Wales to allow therapy support workers to qualify as professional therapists. We were convinced that, given the right training, they could satisfy professional standards. Instead of taking high school leavers with good grades in academic subjects, we would take people, mainly mature ladies, who had left school with few, if any, qualifications. Instead of a full-time diploma course, we would run a part-time programme aimed at people with a wealth of relevant experience but no academic credits. We encountered scepticism and resistance from the profession's headquarters in London. This was not the way they had worked in the past and they had profound reservations about whether standards would be maintained. This was despite our careful research and preparation. It took several years for us to demonstrate that, even though this was not the normal way to train therapists, we could produce staff who provided good-quality care. But, in time, the scheme was seen as a notable success.

Our capacity for persisting with the accepted way of doing things, even when simpler or better ways are available, is remarkable. A common example is the way meetings are run. Even when there is general discontent with meetings that waste time and achieve little, it is still hard to persuade people to leave behind what they know and try a different approach. It is common for team members to endure, sometimes for years, poor meetings without ever raising their concerns in the meeting for fear of criticism. This unwillingness to make the issue discussable virtually guarantees that no changes will even be contemplated, let alone tested.

We also frequently encounter work teams who produce formal minutes for their team meetings, complete with apologies, matters arising, and checking the minutes of the last meeting. All of these things are superfluous for 95% of meetings, not to mention time consuming. Nevertheless, we find that teams are uneasy about not doing what they have always done.

> One persistent fallacy about influencing staff concerns the power of money. Successive large-scale surveys by the City and Guilds organisation in the UK show that high salaries do not lead to satisfying work.[16] Instead, having an interest in what you do was found to be the number one factor in determining happiness at work. Put alongside this the fact that people from all backgrounds voluntarily give their time and effort to charitable causes and we must conclude that the nature of the task and the chance to make a positive difference are more useful than money in influencing behaviour at work.

New ideas and innovations that threaten established practice are often fiercely resisted. The language used in the struggle may be that of logic and scholarly debate but the underlying issue is an attempt to hold onto entrenched assumptions. It's often said that generals are perfectly prepared for fighting the last war by the time the next one comes along, but we can also apply this to organisations. At a time when we need flexibility and innovation, our persistent preoccupation with hierarchy and control is as unsuitable as cavalry charges were in World War I. Many of the ways in which we run teams and organisations are based on assumptions dating back to the Industrial Revolution. Our assumption that fear and greed are the only motivators for change flies in the face of so much evidence that people have been moved by idealism and altruism to learn, innovate and invent.

LEARNING FROM LIFE

It's all too easy to spot how our bosses or colleagues have avoided learning. But before we bemoan the inability of others to learn, we first of all need to turn the spotlight on ourselves. The rest of this chapter aims to help you make sure you are not missing opportunities to learn.

What is called for is a commitment to learning where we take personal responsibility for improving the way we deal with other people, even when the lessons are uncomfortable. And these are lessons which are learned in life, rather than through courses. Research with several professions,[17,18] in the UK and in the USA, shows that informal learning is valued above formal courses and that active approaches such as mentoring, action learning and professional networking are seen as most helpful in continuing professional development. Formal courses, where the learner is largely passive, have their place as a way of providing a basic grounding in essential knowledge and theory, but it seems we learn best when working and learning with others. Particularly in areas that are complex, and where there are few hard-and-fast rules, formal courses are inadequate. Their continuing attraction lies in the fact that large numbers of people can be processed quickly and that the transmission of information can be measured by means of tests or assignments. But acquiring information is not the same as learning, and being able to demonstrate an understanding of theory does not guarantee changes in behaviour. In addition, what universities and colleges want to teach may not be the same as what practitioners want to learn.

TECHNICAL EDUCATION OR PRACTICAL LEARNING?

In his influential study of professional learning, *The Reflective Practitioner*, Donald Schön contrasts the academic world, where problems can be clearly defined, with the day-to-day reality of professional work where issues emerge, mutate and intertwine. He calls this the 'dilemma of rigor or relevance'.[19] 'In the varied topography of professional practice,' Schön argues, 'there is a high, hard ground where practitioners can make effective use of research-based theory and technique, and there is a swampy lowland where situations are confusing "messes" incapable of technical solution. The difficulty is that the problems of the high ground, however great their technical interest, are often relatively unimportant to clients or to the larger society, while in the swamp are the problems of greatest human concern.'

For this reason we have to become what Schön calls reflective practitioners. This requires reflection-on-action, where we review an experience retrospectively in order to learn lessons. But it also requires reflection-in-action (reflexive practice) where we think on our feet and adjust our actions *in the moment* according to what is happening around us. To become effective influencers, we have to unflinchingly review, evaluate and adjust our own actions during and after our encounters with other people. This may seem like a tall order, but the complexities of human behaviour set within the context of organisational culture and politics mean that successful influencing cannot be reduced to a simple formula or set of steps. Instead, we have to actively make sense of this complex area, combining intuition, logic and sound theory.

SUMMARY

We've seen that learning through experience is by no means guaranteed and that we have several very effective ways of defending ourselves from the discomfort that real learning brings. But we can choose to become people who embrace learning rather than people who avoid its challenge. There is, however, a cost. Time and determination are required. The exercises and techniques that follow are intended to enhance your ability to reflect purposefully and to manufacture learning from the raw material of experience.

EXERCISE 1: LEARNING TO LISTEN

One of us was recently coaching a very bright, but very frustrated young professional working in a consultancy firm. 'It's like repeatedly banging your head against a brick wall,' she said, describing her attempts to suggest changes in the way the company ran its projects. Despite a good salary and good working conditions, this talented young lady was rapidly losing motivation because she felt she was not being listened to. Her employers were prepared to pay her well, provide her with an office and all the support she needed, and entrust her with projects worth huge sums of money. But they seemed not to be prepared to listen.

Our experience of consulting to a wide range of organisations in the private, public and voluntary sectors is that much of the time staff do not feel listened to. When we talk to managers about this, their immediate response is that they don't have the time. The implication of this is that listening is a luxury, rightly displaced by more essential tasks. It's a shame that this is such a common point of view, because listening is a powerful tool for problem solving, influencing and, most important of all, making staff feel valued.

Why is listening influential? Partly because by listening carefully to someone, you will set yourself apart from most other people they meet. Regardless of the content of the conversation, just by taking the time to listen you will make a positive impression. Research in the NHS found that staff who felt they were not listened to were more likely to feel demotivated and that those who felt listened to were, not surprisingly, more motivated.[20]

When people feel genuinely listened to, they tend to listen to themselves more carefully. Any reader with experience of working with an interpreter will know that, to help that interpreter convey your words to others, you need to make your speech clear, simple and unambiguous. In other words, you think differently about the words you use. The process is the same when you are truly listening to another person. They will think differently about the words they are using and the issue they are describing. On occasions, merely listening is enough for the other person to solve their own issue.

Listening is particularly important when someone has a complaint to make. Whether they are a member of the public or a colleague, they feel aggrieved and they want that grievance heard and understood. When instead of a listening ear they encounter defensiveness, frustration is added to grievance. This frustration grows as the response they receive is more concerned with not admitting culpability than satisfying someone's need to feel that their point has been taken seriously. Frustration can then become cynicism as the complainant realises how little their view is valued, or even become aggression which will be met with even more defensiveness. In many cases, a readiness to listen can not only avoid such unfortunate consequences, but also enable learning and bridge building between individuals.

We need to learn to listen in a way that is more than just waiting for the other person to stop speaking so we can make our point. This more effective kind of listening is sometimes called active listening, which aims to help someone talk through an issue so as to be able to better understand and manage it. Active listening has the following elements.

➤ **Attending**. Bringing our full attention to bear on what is being said and making this obvious through our body language and by minimising distractions. If we really want to listen, multi-tasking is impossible. Put the phone down, make eye contact, lean forward and nod or grunt to show you are listening.

➤ **Asking open questions**. Asking questions which cannot be answered with a 'yes' or 'no' can help the person explore their situation more fully. These are usually 'why', 'how' and 'who' questions. For instance, if a colleague has a problem with managing his workload, asking 'How do you set priorities?' will elicit more useful information than 'Do you set priorities?'.

➤ **Drawing out**. In response to a statement like 'I'm just no good at managing my time', it's often helpful to invite the person to explain what they mean. Asking questions such as 'Can you tell me more about that?' or 'What leads you to say that?' can lead to the person looking afresh at important issues.

➤ **Summarising/reflecting**. This is where you say back to someone your understanding of what they have told you, e.g. 'So you seem to be saying that working for two people means you are unsure whose work to do first'. This not only allows you to check that you have understood them correctly and demonstrate that you are listening carefully, it also tends to provoke new lines of thinking as they hear their words summarised or paraphrased.

➤ **Suspending judgement**. This means listening with an open mind to allow someone to fully explore or explain an issue. Without this, fresh learning is unlikely for either party because the listener will step in with a solution before they have fully understood the issue and the person being listened to will not have had a chance to develop their own thinking. We regularly find that if we can hold back from trying to solve people's issues for them, they eventually reach solutions for themselves. And even if we do offer some insights or suggestions, they will be better informed than if we had just blundered in with our ideas straight away. This is probably the hardest listening skill for managers and professionals to learn. Their training leads them to want to solve people's problems. For technical issues where there are simple right and wrong answers, this attitude is fine. But the more complex the problem is, the more active listening is called for. In such situations active listening actually trains people to think through and solve their own problems. So although it takes time, skill and patience, it is a good investment. The more we just tell people what they ought to do, the more their own problem-solving skills atrophy.

Listening exercise

In the next few days, when someone wants to explain an issue to you or ask for your help, use active listening. Demonstrate that you are giving them your full attention, suspend judgement and use open questions to help them develop and clarify their own thinking. Good opportunities for active listening include:

➤ when someone comes to you with a complex or recurrent problem
➤ mentoring meetings
➤ appraisal or personal development discussions.

Afterwards, reflect on the conversation and its outcome, both for you and for the other person.

➤ What did you find hard, and why?
➤ What differences from other conversations did you find?
➤ What learning did you gain?

'A KIND OF EPIPHANY'

We teach active listening on several of our programmes and we have heard some remarkable accounts of the way it can change situations which were previously seen as intractable. One manager used it with a member of staff whose domineering behaviour was badly affecting one of her colleagues. She told us that 'having learnt this (active listening) I had the opportunity to use it with the "domineering" person. In what transpired to be a very emotional event, I was able to guide the person towards recognising that her preferred way of expressing her commitment to her role is not the only way of doing so, and that others demonstrate that in other, equally valid ways. Above all, through this process, the member of staff realised that the cause of her anger was not her colleague but a decision taken by another manager. This appeared to lead to a kind of epiphany which led to her going to see the in-house counselling service in order to examine her approach to work and the effect of her behaviour on her relationships with others.'

EXERCISE 2: TEAM LEARNING

This exercise is best done in the context of a team which regularly works together and where there are good levels of honesty and trust. Review the major issues the team has faced in the last few months and try to identify instances where you have unconsciously employed the defences against learning explained in this chapter.

➤ **It's their fault**. This is where we focus on the faults of other people, departments or systems to explain why things went wrong, using this to avoid reflecting on our part in the issue. Do you have people or systems that you habitually blame? Is blaming them taking the focus away from learning or change that your team needs to embrace?

➤ **Something must be done**. This defence against learning involves taking action without sufficient reflection, thereby running the risk of making things worse. What was the biggest challenge or crisis the team faced? What reflection went on before action was taken?

➤ **Treating the symptoms**. This is where the problems we address are just symptoms of deeper issues that we either are unaware of or would prefer to ignore. What recurrent problems or issues do you face? What factors underlie them and are they being addressed?

Make sure the team understands that the aim of the discussion is learning rather than blame. Record any agreements about how the team can avoid these pitfalls in the future.

EXERCISE 3: KEEPING A LEARNING JOURNAL

During a practical session on personal development planning, where we had encouraged people to write down the things in life and work that they really wanted, a participant was talking about why she had found it so helpful. 'I think I knew these things already', she said, 'but writing them down made them more real.' Keeping a learning journal amplifies, clarifies and reflects back to us the learning available to us from daily experience. In the same way that when drawing an object, an artist notices much more about it than if she had just happened to see it in passing, when we write down our recollections and reflections of an incident, we 'see' much more than if we had just thought about them.

Your journal could be a real book or it could be your laptop. As long as it is accessible and confidential, it doesn't matter. There are many ways to keep a journal, but start with the following approach. Choose an experience or situation that surprises, puzzles or interests you, perhaps because it was unexpected or because it went much better or worse than you had anticipated. You could be reflecting on a meeting with a colleague that lasted an hour or on a project that lasted several months. Having selected an experience, make your journal entry in three parts.

1 **Record what happened**. This section is just about what was said, what was done and perhaps what you felt at the time. Be careful to avoid any interpretation or assumptions in this part of your journal entry – stick to the facts.
2 **Reflect on what happened**. Write down your reflections on the experience, focusing on your part in the process. What was going on below the surface? How could you explain what happened? What mental models were at play? How did your actions influence the process?
3 **Learning and planning**. This is where you record the ideas and conclusions that have emerged from your reflection, plus any actions you plan to take as a result.

You will need some self-discipline to get into the habit of making entries in your journal, but once you have established a routine you may well find that it becomes a welcome part of your life, not just making sense of the complex situations you work with but providing a regular opportunity for contemplation and reflection.

ARE YOU READY TO LEARN?

These three exercises will help you become better at turning experience into learning. They will also strengthen you as a positive role model for others. But they all depend on a readiness on our part to admit that we need to learn and change. Such humility is not weakness, it is a source of strength as it keeps our feet firmly on the ground and helps us to avoid hubris – the excessive pride that leads to a fall. Being seen by those around you as someone who is ready to learn and to admit mistakes is, in itself, hugely influential.

REFERENCES

1 IBM Corporation. *Making Change Work*. Somers, NY: IBM Corporation; 2008. www-935.ibm.com/services/us/gbs/bus/html/gbs-making-change-work.html
2 Chief Medical Officer. *An Organisation with a Memory. Report of an expert group on learning from adverse events in the NHS*. London: Stationery Office; 2000. p.4
3 Gregory R, editor. *The Oxford Companion to the Mind*. 2nd ed. Oxford: Oxford University Press; 2004.
4 De Gues A. *The Living Company*. London: Longview; 1997. p.76.
5 Senge P. *The Fifth Discipline*. London: Random House; 1990. p.13.
6 Chapman J. *System Failure*. London: Demos; 2002.
7 Argyris C. Teaching smart people how to learn. *Harvard Bus Rev*. 1991; **May-June**: 99–109.
8 Hamel G. *The Future of Management*. Boston: Harvard Business School Press; 2007. p.53.
9 Ratey J. *A User's Guide to the Brain*. London: Abacus; 2003. The 'Mozart effect' is a good example of the misreporting of research.
10 Semler R. *Maverick*. London: Arrow; 1993. Semler began his radical overhaul of SEMCO in the 1980s. He shocked other industrialists with innovations such as staff selecting their managers. The business is still going strong.
11 Sheldrake J. *Management Theory*. 2nd ed. London: Thomson; 2003.
12 Argyris C. Double-loop learning in organisations. *Harvard Bus Rev*. 1977; **Sept-Oct**: 115–25.
13 Kouzes J, Posner B. *The Leadership Challenge*. 4th ed. San Francisco: Jossey-Bass; 2007. p.122.
14 Ellins J, Ham C. *NHS Mutual: engaging staff and aligning incentives to higher levels of performance*. London: Nuffield Trust; 2009.
15 Ham C. Improving NHS performance. *BMJ*. 1999; **319**(7223): 1490.
16 www.cityandguilds.com/24635.html
17 Cheetham G, Chivers G. How professionals learn in practice: an investigation of informal leaning amongst people working in professions. *J Eur Industr Train*. 2001; 25(5): 247–92.
18 Garet M, Porter A, Desimone L, Birman B, Yoon K. What makes professional development effective? *Am Educ Res J*. 2001; **38**(4): 915–45.
19 Schön D. *The Reflective Practitioner*. London: Temple Smith; 1983. p.42.
20 Finlayson B. *Counting the Smiles: morale and motivation in the NHS*. London: King's Fund; 2002. www.kingsfund.org.uk/publications/ counting_the.html

CHAPTER 2

Learning about yourself

Know thyself.

(Inscription at the Temple of Apollo at Delphi)

Ah wad some power the giftie gie us
To see ourselves as others see us.

(Robert Burns)

In the previous chapter, we explored the process of learning and why we sometimes avoid it. As we turn our attention to you and how you deal with the people around you, bear in mind what we said about defences against learning. These defences work in very subtle ways to preserve our self-image and justify the way we already do things. If you read something that seems to challenge what you know, reflect for a moment before you dismiss it. The ability to do this, to suspend judgement, is essential for the serious learner. Without it, we will miss many an opportunity to change assumptions and opinions that may be outdated or ineffective.

First and foremost, management is about people. It is not a technical exercise, but a human one. Sure, there are technical areas that the wise manager will recognise as important, such as financial management or employment law, but these are secondary and subordinate to the task of building teams of people who willingly give their best in pursuit of the purpose of an enterprise. A good definition of an organisation is a network of people with a purpose. Buildings, equipment and money are all just there to enable the people to achieve their purpose, be it healing the sick, providing public transport or building homes. These resources may be essential but without the people, they are useless. And not just any people will do – they must be motivated, purposeful and well trained. They must be given enough direction for there to be synergy but enough freedom for there to be innovation. They need to be inspired rather than coerced, partners and not just human resources. If they are not, even the biggest budget will not be big enough. Therefore, the manager's primary concern is with people.

LEADERSHIP IS MANAGEMENT PRACTISED WELL

Some people argue that management and leadership are entirely different or even mutually exclusive.[1] Distinctions are made, some simplistic, some well argued, between the manager and the leader. Leaders do the right things, they will say, while managers do things right. Another common view is that leaders develop strategy while managers implement policy. Or, leaders value change, some say, while managers value stability. We find these distinctions unhelpful, not least because of the implication that creativity, innovation and strategy are the province of just a few, probably senior, people called leaders. They also seem to imply that leadership is something which is beyond most people. They reinforce the stereotypes of the heroic, charismatic leader and the faceless, grey-suited manager. We sometimes echo this view of leaders in the way we describe people in organisations. We tend to call junior staff supervisors, administrators or managers, and reserve the term 'leader' for those closer to the boardroom. Not only is this a massive motivational own-goal, but also it unthinkingly underlines the assumption that most staff are just pairs of hands under the direction of senior brains.

MANAGEMENT BAD, LEADERSHIP GOOD?

The management versus leadership debate is a particular issue in the UK National Health Service. In interviews with representatives of 18 professional groups,[2] researchers found that most did not distinguish between management and leadership. The major exception was medicine which, despite being ambiguous about what leadership was, regarded it much more favourably than management. The researchers concluded that many doctors are hostile to the notion of management and suspicious of colleagues who make the transition. Whatever the reasons for this, staff working with doctors may encounter a problem in presenting management as something positive.

We are not the only ones who struggle with this divide between managers and leaders. Henry Mintzberg, Professor of Management at McGill University, who has been researching management since the 1970s, asks whether anyone would like to be managed by someone who couldn't lead or led by someone who couldn't manage. He argues that 'Instead of distinguishing managers from leaders, we should be seeing managers *as* leaders, and leadership as management practiced well'.[3] Others point out that there is no consistent definition of leadership[4] and that what one writer calls leadership, another sees as management.

Distinguishing managers from leaders works better in theory than in practice. If I carry out an appraisal that leaves someone inspired, re-envisioned and with a fresh sense of direction, am I managing or leading? If I make good use of statistics to successfully argue for a radical change in the treatment of dementia, am I managing or leading? Both examples illustrate how, in practice, good leadership usually entails good management and vice versa.

We, along with others, see leadership as a vital part of management which is particularly concerned with motivating people through vision and involvement, but we do not believe that managers and leaders are different sorts of people. Leadership and management overlap, argues Michael Fullan, 'and we need both qualities'.[5]

For these reasons, and for the sake of simplicity, in this book we will not distinguish between managers and leaders or limit management to the application of a set of predetermined tasks. Good leaders manage and good managers lead. From stores administrators and ward managers to chief executives and medical directors, all have the opportunity – we would say duty – to inspire and develop their staff and to push for improvements to the services they deliver. Equally, all have the responsibility to bring order from chaos and make best use of time and money.

THE IMPORTANCE OF SELF-AWARENESS

So if management is primarily about people and, if practised well, includes the things we often call leadership – courage, vision, values and influencing the way people think and act – then a foundation for success is to know yourself, and to understand what sort of manager you are. Carpenters have their tools, artists have brushes and paint and the surgeon has a scalpel, but when it comes to working with people, our only tool is ourselves. For managers, it is who we are and what we know, expressed in our words and actions, that matter. As we noted above, there are many useful technical skills we can develop, but these have a supporting role. In fact, it is an over-reliance on techniques as opposed to hard-won wisdom that gets many graduates of Masters in Business Administration (MBA) programmes a bad press. Such programmes provide aspiring managers with a wealth of techniques for analysis and decision making, which, not surprisingly, they then attempt to use in the real world. The trouble is, instead of human resources, they encounter real people.

Dov Frohman, brilliant innovator and manager at Intel, speaks for many when he argues that leadership cannot be taught, but it can be learned.[6] Mastery of every technique for analysis and decision making is of little use if we have not mastered our primary management tool – ourselves. To do this, we need to know what we're good at, how we come across, and what our flaws and biases might be. In short, we need to be self-aware.

MANAGING WITHOUT CONTROLLING

Most of the managers we work with tell us that one of their greatest challenges is how to manage people whom they cannot control or coerce. These might be colleagues, people senior to them or people who work in other organisations, but without their co-operation progress is difficult or impossible. In such circumstances self-awareness is critical. Simply telling people what to do is counterproductive even with staff who report to you, but with those who do not, it is potentially disastrous. We must rely on our ability to influence without power, and this in turn depends on how others see us and whether we are respected and trusted. A manager who lacks self-awareness in these situations is about as useful as a workman who arrives at your house with no idea what tools are in his bag.

TO SEE OURSELVES AS OTHERS SEE US

The importance of self-awareness is underlined by research into the way managers assess themselves compared with how they are rated by their colleagues. Overall, these studies show that effective managers tend to rate themselves very similarly to the way others rate them. For example, one study found that those managers who under-rated themselves or rated themselves similarly to the way others rated them were identified as the most effective by their followers.[7] It seems that effective managers have a more realistic view of themselves, having achieved what Robert Burns could only wish for and seeing themselves as others see them. Far from trying to protect a fragile self-image, they actually seek out negative feedback.

In contrast, poorly performing managers have an unrealistically favourable view of themselves compared with the way their colleagues see them.[8-10]

CEO DISEASE

Daniel Goleman coined this phrase to describe the paradox that it is those people who most need good, honest feedback – those in very senior positions – who are least likely to receive it. For a mixture of reasons, including fear of reprisals, people around those occupying top jobs will often withhold negative feedback. In the absence of accurate feedback, senior people must fall back on their own self-perception. But here's the worst part of CEO disease: it is the poorest performers who over-rate their capabilities the most.[11]

Daniel Goleman sees self-awareness as one of the main components of emotional intelligence, or EQ. He argues that mere IQ is not enough, particularly when it comes to dealing with other people. We have probably all met people who are bright and well qualified but who are a liability in sensitive interpersonal situations. Often they seem blissfully unaware of the impact they are having, unable to see what is obvious to others – when to speak, when to listen, when to press a point and when to hold back. Such people will always be limited in their effectiveness whatever their professional qualifications. On the other hand, we also encounter people who just seem to know how to get the best from others, dealing with disgruntled staff or distressed members of the public with a skill that they were not taught and could not explain. The empathy, self-awareness and self-control exhibited in such situations are the result of emotional intelligence. Disciplines such as psychology can dissect and describe this behaviour in theoretical terms but it cannot be acquired through theory.

In his book *The New Leaders*, Goleman helpfully divides self-awareness into three aspects.[11]

➤ Emotional self-awareness
➤ Accurate self-assessment
➤ Self-confidence

These three facets of self-awareness lie at the heart of effective management. Without them, we are unlikely to be able to deal with anything but the most technical parts of the management task. Let's take a moment to think about ourselves in relation to these three areas.

Emotional self-awareness

The self-aware manager understands his emotions and the impact they have on his performance. For those who see management as a largely technical exercise, where logic is applied to quantifiable issues in order to make decisions, emotions may seem irrelevant. But whether or not we approve of emotion in the workplace, a moment's reflection will confirm the inevitability of an emotional component to any human interaction. We come to work as whole people, complete with emotions as well as hands and brains. So every time we interact with one another, communication is happening on several levels: verbal and non-verbal, rational and emotional, conscious and intuitive. Objective logic is an essential management tool, but it takes more than logic to influence people. Factors such as loyalty, hope and enthusiasm all have a profound impact on how we work and are unlikely to be inspired by rational arguments alone.

Acknowledging and understanding this emotional dimension of management is part of self-awareness. Being able to deal with our own and others' emotions, what we might call emotional literacy, is a huge asset, whereas denying the importance or even existence of this dimension of organisational life seriously limits our ability to lead and to influence.

EI AT SEA: THE IMPACT OF THE MANAGER'S MOOD

In an innovative study which looked at the leadership behaviours of skippers in a round-the-world yacht race,[12] the emotional intelligence of the skippers was assessed and rated during the race using interviews with the skippers and their crews. Overall, a relationship between emotional intelligence and high performance was found. One skipper, rated low to medium, seemed unaware of the impact his emotional moods had on the crew. After a tactical decision went wrong, he retired to his bunk, and he was described as being unable to control his feelings towards people he did not like or respect. Another skipper, rated more highly for emotional intelligence, was described by a crew member thus: 'In a crisis he is calm and collected and created confidence in the crew, who respond well and maintain their performance'. The message is clear. Good managers understand the impact their moods have on those around them and have the self-control needed to make sure the impact is positive.

Goleman also sees intuition as part of emotional self-awareness. From Chester Barnard,[13] writing in the 1930s, to current researchers such as Claxton, many have argued that good managers use intuition in decision making, particularly where the issue is complex and the number or nature of the factors involved rules out explicit analysis. The self-aware manager is comfortable using intuition, but deliberately balances it with logic and objectivity. In fast-changing situations where much that is important is unknown or only partly understood, deductive logic cannot function but intuition thrives.

Healthcare managers often need to reach decisions or make plans where information is incomplete and where the actions of the other staff or agencies involved cannot be predicted with any confidence. One response to this is to obsessively collect more and more data as if sheer volume could overcome the complexity of the situation. But this can lead to paralysis by analysis or, just as dangerously, the delusion that the future can be predicted. This applies particularly to strategy making, where 'well-developed, tentatively used intuition is actually the best tool for the job; while the apparent solidity of a rational strategic plan offers nothing more than a comforting illusion'.[14]

In a piece of research one of us carried out with top managers from the public sector, several of them said that they consciously incorporated intuition into their decision making.[15] One told us how, when faced with a particularly complex decision, he had gone through all the available information but deliberately not reached a conclusion until he had slept on it. On waking the next morning, it was as though he had processed the issue whilst asleep. His mind was now clearer and he was able to make a decision he was comfortable with.

Self-aware managers also have a strong sense of their own priorities and values which then guides their decisions. Rather than being blown this way and that by circumstances, they pursue long-term goals which reflect deeply held convictions. As part of one of our programmes, we ask managers to consider how close they are to achieving their life goals. In the discussion that follows, most will admit that they do not have clear goals beyond their immediate situation. They are consumed by the present demands of work and family. While this is very understandable, it is also a cause for concern. They run the risk of reaching the end of their career with the basic question of life purpose unanswered. To begin to answer questions of this magnitude takes time and space. To be emotionally aware requires thoughtful, unhurried reflection. Some might call this prayer or meditation, and in the previous chapter we encouraged you to use a learning journal to aid such reflection, but however we do it, regular reflection provides a place where a sense of our own identity and purpose can form. It is this clarifying of who we are and where we are going in life that helps us keep a sense of perspective in trying times.

ARE YOU A SERVANT-LEADER?

In recent years there has been increasing interest in the concept of servant-leadership. Although Greenleaf first coined the term in the 1970s, it resonates strongly with the aspirations and concerns of many leaders today. Instead of seeing people as resources to be exploited in pursuit of short-term gains, the servant-leader seeks to build learning communities which use resources wisely. Instead of seeing leadership as a chance to look good or further their own reputation, the servant-leader regards it as an opportunity to serve, through good leadership, their staff and the wider community. Servant-leadership is not a quick fix or a technique but a set of values that affect every aspect of the leader's thought and action.

Among the characteristics of the servant-leader are self-awareness, empathy, the ability to listen and the use of persuasion rather than hierarchical authority. But the best test is whether you are committed to the growth of the people you work with. To quote Greenleaf: 'Do those served grow as persons; do they, while being served, become healthier, wiser, freer, more autonomous, more likely themselves to become servants?'.[16] This is a tough question for any leader but one which, in our view, is worth serious reflection.

Are you a servant-leader?

Accurate self-assessment

Earlier in this chapter we considered the link between good management and a realistic self-assessment. It seems that good managers not only accept feedback, they actually go looking for it! Through reflecting unflinchingly on such feedback, they know where they are strong and where they are weak. The quiet confidence that this engenders is a world away from the attitude, born of machismo, that sees admitting weakness as a failure. Believing that we can be successful at everything is unrealistic and will lead to disappointment as we over-reach ourselves. The antidote is not self-denigration but accurate self-assessment, which acknowledges both strengths and weaknesses. Knowing our strengths is essential if we are to play to them and knowing our weaknesses helps us to know when to seek help or to let others take the lead. It is not that we should do ourselves down or become apologetic every time we are in the limelight; this is as harmful as being overconfident. It is more a recognition that each of us has a unique set of strengths or gifts, but that no one is gifted in every area. This enables us to be secure in our self-worth and this security in turn enables us to admit that we have much still to learn.

Self-confidence

When we can accept ourselves for who we are, celebrating our strengths and acknowledging our weaknesses, we have self-confidence. Not bravado, which is brittle, but a solid belief in our abilities based on feedback and reflection. Armed with this, we can meet new challenges without fear. We know where we are strong and we know where we will need support. This unflappable confidence does not only affect our personal contribution, it also inspires our colleagues. In the same way that panic seems to be infectious, spreading nervousness and frantic activity, so confidence affects those around us. In difficult times we can be powerfully influential just by displaying confidence and refusing to lose perspective. If we lead a team, our confidence will spill over to our colleagues. Teamwork can only function when we make room for one another's gifts, and this requires confidence not only in what we can do but also in the abilities of our team-mates. In fact, an honest but supportive team is a great place to learn self-confidence as we recognise each other's contribution.

BUILDING SELF-AWARENESS

So how can we become more self-aware? Thankfully, there are several ways in which we can obtain useful information about ourselves. In fact, getting the information is relatively easy; the hard part is accepting and acting upon it!

Self-reflection

We've put this first because being prepared to spend some time thinking honestly and deeply about yourself and how you affect others is the starting point for all that follows. Our minds may be busy all day long, but the depth and focus of our thoughts are hampered by the myriad distractions we encounter. When we are thinking in a hurry, our minds are likely to slip into familiar paths, making fresh insights difficult. If we are continually rushing from task to task or from one form of entertainment to another, we may be unaware of deeper currents of thought and emotion. Sometimes these thoughts, insights and decisions take time to bubble up to the surface. Guy Claxton calls this 'slow knowing' and he contrasts it with the frantic pace in some organisations where 'meetings proliferate; the working day expands; time gets shorter. So much time is spent processing information, solving problems and meeting deadlines that there is none left in which to think'.[14]

Some time ago, a nurse came to a session we ran on personal development. For the first time in many years, she was given time to think about herself and what she really wanted from her career. As she considered the questions we asked her, she slowly became aware that although she was rising up through her professional hierarchy, she was not happy in her work. As she reflected further, she realised that what really satisfied her was direct patient care and that, on consideration, this was more important to her than promotion. She had been given time and opportunity for something she knew at a deep level to come to the surface and she was able to reshape her career as a result. Her story is just one of many where more sustained reflection has led first to deeper insight and then to positive change.

If your work resembles a merry-go-round of endless information, pressing demands and stress-tinged conversations, it is vital that you find time to reflect. It will help you distinguish progress from mere activity and restore your sense of perspective. By making time for 'slow knowing', your awareness of who you are, what's important to you and where you're going will increase. One busy clinician we know always takes one week each year as a silent retreat. Initially the change of pace is difficult, but she finds the experience profoundly restorative and returns to the task of running her department with freshness and energy. Another manager interviewed by one of us, who has a consistent track record of innovation and relentless optimism, attributes his energy and insight to his daily session of contemplative prayer and reading.

The kind of insights that come from reflection or 'slow knowing' cannot be preplanned or organised. Instead, we need to create times when such thoughts can slowly take shape and become conscious. From Archimedes to recent Nobel Prize winners,[17] many profound insights come precisely when we are *not* consciously thinking about them. The time you spend walking along the beach or staring at the fire may well be more productive in terms of self-reflection than labouring with the issue in your office. So put some time aside for reflection. A walk in the country perhaps, away from the demands of home and office. If you need a loose structure for your thoughts, try these three questions: What am I grateful for? How would I know my life had been successful? What would I want my legacy to be?

Feedback from others: 'How am I doing?'

A suggestion we often make to managers is that they should ask their staff: 'How am I doing?'. Although the initial reaction may be stunned silence, we guarantee, provided they believe you want an honest answer, that you will receive useful feedback. Staff may be reluctant to give you an honest response. This could be because their experience of organisations tells them to filter out anything that could be deemed critical (see 'CEO disease' above). It could also be because they tried giving feedback to a previous boss, or even to you, and felt rebuffed. As well as giving feedback to your staff, try asking them for feedback on how they are being managed and how you could manage them more effectively. The 360° appraisal, where several people who work with you use a questionnaire to anonymously rate your performance in different skills areas, provides a way round the reluctance of some to give honest feedback. It also enables quantitative comparisons between the various raters and your own self-assessment. However, it should be seen as a complement to, rather than a replacement for, face-to-face dialogue.

Such feedback, from those prepared to give it, is worth its weight in gold. Listen carefully and, most importantly, resist the urge to defend or justify yourself. Once we are focusing on explaining why we were right, the opportunity for learning is lost.

HOW WOULD YOU LIKE TO BE MANAGED?

Our best case studies come from our many and frequent mistakes. One of us, early in his management career, was successful in getting a star performer transferred to his team. Her reputation was that of administrative goddess: calm, efficient and confident. But soon after joining my team, she became unhappy and her performance began to decline. The reason? I had been managing her as I liked to be managed, giving her a few long-term goals and adopting a very hands-off style. But what she wanted was to work to very explicit performance targets and to review them, with her boss, each week. Once I had found this out and started to manage her differently, her performance improved again. If I had just asked her how she wanted to be managed at the start of our relationship, I could have saved her, and myself, a large amount of trouble. Instead, I had assumed that my preferences were everyone's preferences and that I knew how people should be managed – a staggering lack of self-awareness.

How long since your last appraisal?

We routinely ask our course participants to tell us how long it has been since they had a meaningful appraisal discussion with their boss, one where the communication was two-way and the outcome was a good understanding of how they were performing and how they and their work might develop in the future. Initially we were shocked by the number of people who reported that several years had passed since such an event but now, having heard so many such stories, these tales of organisational malpractice only sadden rather than surprise us.

Appraisal is a well-researched and simple way to improve teams and organisations. It takes a little time and thought, but the results outweigh the effort. Finding managers who do not appraise their staff is a little like finding a doctor who refuses to use antibiotics. There is a proven strong relationship between good appraisal and job satisfaction[18] and in a study of hospitals in England, the 'extent and sophistication of appraisal systems in hospitals was closely related to lower mortality rates'.[19] So, before organisations look for the latest ways of motivating or developing their staff, they should first check that appraisal is being done – and done well – at all levels. It deepens communication, clarifies roles and goals and motivates staff. As our American friends say, it is a 'no brainer'.

One of the great benefits of having an appraisal is the opportunity it provides for us to become more self-aware. Sure, your boss's view will be flawed. Their position and prejudices will mean that they will notice some things and fail to see others. But even with these distortions, we can learn much from a well-delivered appraisal. If your boss is nervous or inexperienced, you can help them by suggesting that the discussion covers these three areas.

➤ Your performance over the last 6–12 months, in terms of both meeting your objectives and your personal contribution to the team.

➤ Suitable goals or targets for the next 6–12 months.

➤ The support or training you will need to reach these goals.

Both you and your boss should come prepared with thoughts and suggestions based on these areas. Other questions you could explore with your boss include:

➤ How do your goals fit in to those of the wider team or organisation?

➤ What are your longer term development goals and aspirations and how could your boss facilitate these?

Many managers have received no training in how to give an appraisal, and their own experiences may have led them to see it as an ordeal rather than an opportunity, so it is not surprising that they avoid carrying out appraisals. Taking the initiative to ask them to give you feedback and gently suggesting a structure like the one above will make it easier and more productive for both of you. If you feel more guidance would be helpful, we say more about appraisal in another book, *Essential Skills for Managing in Healthcare*.[20]

Take a test!

Psychometric tests can be another good way to gain insight into yourself and how other people see you. Both of us use personality tests as part of our coaching and career development work, and we frequently find that they provide clients with much greater self-understanding. We have found the following tests helpful in our work.

➤ **Myers–Briggs Type Indicator (MBTI)**. We'll say more about this later in the chapter.

➤ **Cattell's 16PF**. A test designed to measure the personality dimensions that affect a person's behaviour.

➤ **California Personality Inventory (CPI)**. A measure of professional and personal styles.

➤ **Belbin Self-Perception Inventory**. This focuses on our behaviour in a team context.

Most tests can only be administered and interpreted by an appropriately qualified practitioner, so make sure that whoever you ask to provide these tests is suitably trained.

PEOPLE ARE DIFFERENT: THE MYERS–BRIGGS TYPE INDICATOR

If management is primarily a human rather than technical process, then the sort of person you are will play an important part in shaping how you manage. And particularly when it comes to influencing, personality plays a major role in determining both the process and the outcome. We'll use the Myers–Briggs Type Indicator (MBTI) to explore the role personality plays, but the essential lesson is this: people are different. Organisations are slowly getting better at acknowledging the impact of obvious differences such as age, gender and skin colour but difference goes beyond what can be observed. Our personality influences how we respond to others to the extent that an approach that works well with one person may completely backfire with another. So just because differences in personality are much less apparent than, say, differences in age or national culture, we should not fall into the trap of ignoring them.

Some years ago, one of us had to deal with a situation where communication between two senior staff had broken down. They had been working together to design a training programme and, as usual, Steve had come with his ideas very carefully prepared but he presented them in his characteristically understated way. Kate, who liked to do her thinking on the spot and who loved nothing better than some verbal sparring, happily tore into his proposals. Steve was deeply offended. He had spent hours developing his ideas and took exception to the way Kate just ripped them apart with no acknowledgement of his hard work. But being Steve, he said nothing of this, instead becoming more and more withdrawn and saying less and less. Through Kate's eyes, this looked like lack of interest and in her frustration, she argued and challenged even more to try and draw Steve into the sort of energetic debate she preferred. And of course, the more Kate provoked, the more Steve withdrew. Further meetings followed a similar pattern until the project ground to a halt.

It took a lengthy meeting with a colleague acting as mediator to bring them to a place where they understood that no malice or disrespect was intended on either side. Both Kate and Steve had been trying to work in the way they preferred to work and not making any allowances for each other. Steve was reserved and quite sensitive, preferring to discuss things in a very calm and thoughtful way. Kate was very outgoing and spontaneous and thrived on passionate, high-decibel debate. Each interpreted the other's behaviour in the light of their own preferences. In other words, Kate saw Steve's understated style as evidence that he had no strong views and saw his withdrawal as an unwillingness to co-operate rather than as the consequence of her own behaviour. Steve saw Kate's enthusiastic debating as aggressive, and as evidence that she had no respect for him or his ideas. The unconscious assumption they had both made was one many managers are guilty of: everyone is like me ... or jolly well ought to be!

But we are not all the same. We have different preferences about how we work, how we communicate and a host of other things. And what is more, these differences are to be celebrated rather than bemoaned. In innovative teams, it is the differences in how we see an issue that lead to new ideas. We need the shoot-from-the-hip types as much as the quiet ones who don't say much but do a lot of thinking. We need the detail guys as much as the big picture visionaries. We need passion and we need logic. But what makes it possible to weave different approaches together into a potent synergy is a readiness to see that people really are different, and that it is a good thing that they are!

We regularly use the MBTI to help people understand their personality preferences and to see how they differ from other personality types. In this chapter we'll give you an overview of the MBTI and invite you to use it to reflect on your personality and how this affects the way you manage and, in particular, how you influence people.

Background

The MBTI addresses the fact that many people with whom we come into contact do not think as we do, value the same things or see the world in the way we see it. The theory underpinning the MBTI suggests that much of this 'seemingly chance variation in human behaviour is not due to chance; it is in fact the logical result of a few basic, observable differences in mental functioning'.[21]

The MBTI sets out four types of differences and the questionnaire allows you to assess your preferences in each type, or dimension, of difference. The four dimensions are as follows.

➤ **Extraversion or Introversion**, which is concerned with where you focus your attention and what energises you.

➤ **Sensing or Intuition**, which is concerned with what kind of information you pay attention to and how you acquire information.

➤ **Thinking or Feeling**, which is about how you prefer to make decisions.

➤ **Judging or Perceiving**, which is about the lifestyle you prefer.

Preference

According to MBTI theory, each of us will have a preference for one of the two opposites in each dimension. For example, you may prefer extraversion to introversion. However, no matter how clear your preference for extraversion is, there may be times when you behave more like an introvert. In MBTI terms, your personality type is a preference, not a straitjacket.

In MBTI literature,[22] this idea of preference is often illustrated by the concept of 'handedness'. In other words, although we tend to use one hand much more than the other for writing or for work that demands precision, we still have two hands and can use both. Nevertheless, we are generally more comfortable and skilled when using our preferred hand. Similarly, although we will have consistent preferences in terms of personality, we may occasionally act outside them. But we will tend to be more comfortable and at our best when acting in line with our preferences. Try writing something with your 'wrong' hand. You'll probably feel clumsy, and the writing may well look quite childish. It also seems to take more concentration and energy to write what, with our preferred hand, we would normally have dashed off without much thought. But whilst those who are right handed will struggle to write with their left hand, for others the left hand is their preference. This is a good way of illustrating differences in personality. Each person will have preferences for how they deal with people and the world in general, which to them seem natural. These are not conscious choices. Instead, like being right or left handed, they seem to be innate. But they will differ from person to person, and what is natural and comfortable for one may be uncomfortable for another.

Let me illustrate this from my own experience. Many years ago, I (AP) accompanied my boss, Professor Stephen Prosser, to a conference in The Netherlands where we had been asked to present a paper we had co-written. The conference began with a very grand reception in the town hall where several hundred academics from all over Europe were gathering, almost all of them strangers to us. On entering the room, Stephen quickly began to start introducing himself to different groups, exchanging business cards and occasionally arranging to meet later during the conference. I, however, after a few half-hearted attempts to join conversations, headed for the buffet table and the free literature and sat in a quiet corner until the ordeal was over. Stephen had acted in line with his Extravert preferences. Meeting new people and making new connections was something that energised him and that he was comfortable with. He needed no pressure or encouragement to strike up conversations and would have felt awkward if he had not been able to do so. On the other hand, my preference for Introversion meant that the very thing that energised Stephen, I found draining and uncomfortable. Trying to strike up a conversation with people I did not know made me feel self-conscious and awkward, like writing with the wrong hand. Over time, I managed to improve my networking skills but it was never something that came naturally to me. Even when I became more skilled, I never wanted to spend too much time in informal situations with people I knew little or not at all.

As we go through each of the four sets of preferences, we'll invite you to self-assess and decide which one of each pair describes you best. While you'll find this useful, it's not a substitute for completing the MBTI questionnaire and having one-to-one feedback from a qualified practitioner. You'll get even more benefit from individual feedback, particularly if you find it hard to identify your preferences from the descriptions that follow. Your personnel department should be able to put you in touch with an MBTI practitioner.

Extraversion (E)	Introversion (I)
Where do you prefer to focus your attention? How are you energised? Which description more closely reflects your preference?	
Preference to draw your energy from the world around you, from 'doing', from involvement in external events and contact with people	Preference to draw your energy from your internal world, through quiet reflection, focusing on your inner thoughts or ideas
• Attuned to external environment	• Drawn to contemplation in inner world
• Prefer to 'talk through' problems	• Prefer to 'think through' problems
• Learn best through doing or discussing	• Learn best by reflection, mental 'practice'
• Breadth of interests	• Depth of interests
• Tend to speak and act first, reflect later	• Tend to reflect before acting or speaking

If the description on the left fits you best, then your preference is likely to be Extraversion (E). If the one on the right describes you more closely, your preference is probably Introversion (I). You may see aspects of yourself on both sides of the line and consequently find it hard to choose. But remember that this is about preference and that your MBTI type is not a straitjacket. If you read through both descriptions again you'll probably find that, overall, one side fits better than the other. The following examples may also help you to clarify your preference.

➤ Introverts often prefer to communicate in writing. Two Introverts who worked in the same office area would frequently email each other rather than talk.

➤ Extraverts often welcome distractions and interruptions. One Extravert we know, when moving to a new, open plan office, deliberately placed her desk between the door and the drinks machine where she thought most people would pass close by.

➤ Introverts and Extraverts, after a draining day, often choose to 'recharge their batteries' in different ways. Introverts may go 'inwards' by reading or listening to music whereas Extraverts may focus 'outwards' by going out or meeting friends.

➤ Introverts do much of their thinking on the inside and Extraverts often like to develop ideas in conversation with others. So when each type presents an idea they may well be at different stages in the thought process. For the Extravert, it could be just an opening gambit intended to spark discussion. For the Introvert it might well be a carefully considered conclusion.

Sensing (S)	Intuition (N)
What kind of information do you prefer to pay attention to? How do you acquire information? Which description more closely reflects your preference?	
Preference for attending to specific information and facts to find out what is actually happening. Observant of what is going on around you and especially focused on the practical realities of the situation	Preference for attending to the patterns and associations between facts rather than the facts themselves. Interested in connections and looking for what might be rather than what is, focusing on ideas and possibilities
• Focus on what is real and actual	• Focus on 'big picture' possibilities
• Value practical applications	• Value imaginative insights
• Factual and concrete, notice details	• Abstract and theoretical
• Observe and remember specifics	• See patterns and meanings in facts
• Enjoy the present	• Enjoy anticipating the future
• Want information to be accurate and precise	• Stimulated by ambiguity
• Trust experience	• Trust inspiration

Again, use the descriptions to self assess. And as with Extraversion and Introversion, you may well see yourself on both sides of the line. But try and identify whether your overall preference is for Sensing (S) or Intuition (N). Here are some more examples of Sensing and Intuitive behaviour.

➤ When travelling with a Sensing companion, an Intuitive noticed that during gaps between flights, his companion would often use his time to explore a city nearby whereas he himself would wait impatiently for the next flight. His Intuitive preference meant that he tended to be focused on the future – in this case the next leg of the journey – whereas his Sensing companion was more focused on what could be done in the present.

➤ We've noticed that, when asked to give travel directions, people with a Sensing preference tend to give precise, detailed information ('go to the second set of lights, turn left and go through another set of lights, then turn right at the garage ...') whereas Intuitives tend to struggle to be specific, even though they know the way.

➤ The 1992 Mike Myers film *Wayne's World* provided a humorous illustration of the difference between Sensing and Intuition. The Mike Myers character, although practically penniless, would routinely drool over a very expensive guitar in a shop window and tell himself 'It will be mine, O yes, it will be mine'. His friend, expressing the tendency of many Sensors to be practical and realistic, would sigh and say 'Live in the now, Wayne, you'll never afford it'. Intuitives tend to live, as it were, in the future, whereas Sensors tend to be focused on the present.

➤ A coaching client with a preference for Intuition found the MBTI helpful in understanding sources of tension with some of his Board colleagues. He would often make suggestions for future developments based on intuitive leaps. The Sensors on the board would struggle with this, preferring to be able to reason their way, step by step, from where they were to where they were going. To them, his ideas seemed to come out of left field rather than being based on concrete facts.

Thinking (T)	Feeling (F)
How do you prefer to make decisions? Which description more closely fits your preference?	
Preference for making decisions from a detached standpoint, by analysing the logical consequences of a choice or action. Applying objective criteria and using consistent rules and principles. Often trying to stand outside a situation to examine it objectively and analyse cause and effect • Guided by objective logic • Focus on cause and effect • Look for flaws in logic • Apply consistent principles in dealing with people • At work, emphasise involvement with tasks	Preference for making decisions from an involved standpoint, by gauging the impact of actions on your personal convictions. Seeking harmony and judging the importance of the different values involved. Often placing yourself inside a situation so as to identify personally with its key values • Guided by personal values and convictions • Focus on harmony with own and others' values • Look for common ground and shared values • Treat each person as a unique individual • At work, emphasise and support the process

In our experience, many health professionals find assessing themselves on this dimension particularly hard. It could be that their training as clinicians teaches them to address problems logically and objectively, using a classic scientific approach. This may lead them to see Thinking as the right way to make decisions, regardless of their natural preference. This view of objective logic as the only correct way to reach a decision is prevalent in many organisations and professions. Perhaps because of this, some clients with a Feeling preference tell us that they still reach conclusions guided primarily by Feeling but that they express these conclusions in the Thinking 'language' which is more readily accepted by their colleagues. In other words, having made up their minds guided by empathy and values, they will present their conclusion using the language of option appraisal and dispassionate analysis.

A helpful way to see the relationship of Thinking and Feeling in decision making is to remember that we can all use both of them in making decisions but that our preference will be the one we use first. So someone with a Thinking preference, when faced with a decision, will first tend to use objective logic to analyse the issue and generate options. But he can then use Feeling to consider these options in the light of his values and the potential impact on people. Someone with a Feeling preference might do the opposite, using Feeling to decide what to do, but then using Thinking to test out their decision. It may help to put aside everyday understandings of the two words. In MBTI theory, both Thinking and Feeling are rational processes that can lead to good decisions but they work from very different perspectives.

➤ A friend with a Thinking preference once made a list of attributes that her future husband must possess. Although she joked about the list, it was noticeable, when she married some years later, how close to her original criteria her husband was.

➤ One of us (with a preference for Feeling) had a successful work partnership with someone with a Thinking preference. In tackling difficult staff issues, she would helpfully remind me of the principles involved to stop me being overwhelmed by more subjective factors. In turn, I would help her consider the individuals we were dealing with, and their unique values and personality.

➤ Both preferences are concerned with fairness. For someone with a Thinking preference, fairness may be about treating people equally or consistently. For someone with a Feeling preference, to be fair is to treat each person as a unique individual.

➤ In examining proposals, people with a Thinking preference will tend to focus first on spotting flaws in the decision-making process whereas those with a Feeling preference may focus first on how the proposals will affect the people involved.

Judging (J)	Perceiving (P)

Which lifestyle do you prefer?
Which description more closely reflects your preference?

Judging (J)	Perceiving (P)
Preference for coming to closure on decisions, preferring to live life in scheduled and orderly ways and wanting things to be controlled and regulated. Liking to make plans and then sticking to those plans until they are completed. Getting satisfaction from getting things done • Like to get things decided • Scheduled and organised • Enjoy decision making and planning • Dislike working under time pressure	Preference for keeping open to new experiences and information. Preferring to live life in a flexible, spontaneous way. Comfortable going with the flow and taking advantage of last-minute options as they arise. Enjoying using resourcefulness and adaptability, and feeling constrained by plans and structures • Like to keep options open • Spontaneous and adaptable • Enjoy the process, no decision before its time • Energised by last-minute pressures

Based on the description above, do you see your preference as Judging (J) or Perceiving (P)? Remember that it is your overall preference that we are trying to clarify. Most people, whatever their preference, want some order and some flexibility. If you're not sure, the following examples may help.

➤ Sally was an excellent project manager with a Judging preference. She systematically organised each project into a series of tasks and deadlines which she then proceeded to accomplish one by one, usually with time to spare. Working with either of us (we both have a preference for Perceiving) was a challenge for her as we tended to start the project with a burst of enthusiasm but then leave most of the work until the final deadline was imminent. Despite the last-minute rush, we would normally finish inside the deadline, just! Both types understand the importance of deadlines, but use them in different ways.

➤ One of us worked for a boss with a Perceiving preference. He loved using his considerable intelligence to generate ideas and options. On one occasion he asked me to come up with three options for tacking a particular issue. I proceeded to take the options to him but when I left his office, instead of a decision, I had three more options!

➤ For many people who prefer Judging, the desire to live an organised life extends into their leisure time, whereas for people with a Perceiving preference, part of the attraction of having time off is the idea that it is 'free' time, unconstricted and full of possibility. We know of couples, one with a preference for Judging and the other with a preference for Perceiving, who find this a source of tension when planning holidays together. The one with a

Judging preference will tend to want to plan activities in advance whereas the other would prefer to 'just get there and see how we feel'.

➤ A hospital manager, whose job involved frequently being asked for decisions by a range of staff, found the MBTI helpful in identifying why he needed to move on. It was not that the decisions were too complex or intellectually challenging, it was more that his preference for Perceiving made him uncomfortable in a role which was all about closing down options rather than generating them. As a result, he found the work draining.

Your four-letter type

Hopefully, the descriptions and examples above will have enabled you to decide whether you prefer:

➤ Extraversion or Introversion (E or I)
➤ Sensing or Intuition (S or N)
➤ Thinking or Feeling (T or F)
➤ Judging or Perceiving (J or P).

Record your self-assessment in the box below, putting a circle around your chosen preference in each pair of preferences.

E or I   S or N   T or F   J or P

Putting together the letters you have circled will give you a four-letter type, e.g. ISFJ or ENTP. This is your 'self-assessed' type. Sixteen different types are possible, and the box below shows some of the characteristics frequently associated with each type. Read through the one that matches your four-letter type and see if it fits your view of yourself.

Characteristics frequently associated with each type

ISTJ

Serious, quiet, earn success by concentration and thoroughness. Practical, orderly, matter-of-fact, logical, realistic and dependable. See to it that everything is well organised. Take responsibility. Make up their own minds as to what should be accomplished and work towards it steadily, regardless of protests or distractions

ISFJ

Quiet, friendly, responsible, and conscientious. Work devotedly to meet their obligations. Lend stability to any project or group. Thorough, painstaking, accurate. Their interests are not usually technical. Can be patient with necessary details. Loyal, considerate, perceptive, concerned with how other people feel

ISTP

Cool onlookers – quiet, reserved, observing and analysing life with detached curiosity and unexpected flashes of original humour. Usually interested in cause and effect, how and why mechanical things work, and in organising facts using logical principles. Excel at getting to the core of a practical problem and finding the solution

ESTP

Good at on-the-spot problem solving. Like action, enjoy whatever comes along. Tend to like mechanical things and sports. Adaptable, tolerant, pragmatic; focused on getting results. Dislike long explanations. Are best with real things that can be worked, handled, taken apart, or put together

ESTJ

Practical, realistic, matter-of-fact, with a natural head for business or mechanics. Not interested in abstract theories; want learning to have direct and immediate application. Like to organise and run activities. Often make good administrators; are decisive, quickly move to implement decisions; take care of routine details

INFJ

Succeed by perseverance, originality, and desire to do whatever is needed or wanted. Put their best efforts into their work. Quietly forceful, conscientious, concerned for others. Respected for their firm principles. Likely to be honoured and followed for their clear visions as to how best to serve the common good

INFP

Quiet observers, idealistic, loyal. Important that outer life be congruent with inner values. Curious, quick to see possibilities, often serve as catalysts to implement ideas. Adaptable, flexible and accepting unless a value is threatened. Want to understand people and ways of fulfilling human potential. Little concern with possessions or surroundings

ISFP

Retiring, quietly friendly, sensitive, kind, modest about their abilities. Shun disagreements, do not force their opinions or values on others. Usually do not care to lead but are often loyal followers. Often relaxed about getting things done because they enjoy the present moment and do not want to spoil it by undue haste or exertion

ESFP

Outgoing, accepting, friendly, enjoy everything and make things more fun for others by their enjoyment. Like action and making things happen. Know what's going on and join in eagerly. Find remembering facts easier than mastering theories. Are best in situations that need sound common sense and practical ability with people

ESFJ

Warm-hearted, talkative, popular, conscientious, born co-operators, active committee members. Need harmony and may be good at creating it. Always doing something nice for someone. Work best with encouragement and praise. Main interest is in things that directly and visibly affect people's lives

INTJ

Have original minds and great drive for their own ideas and purposes. Have long-range vision and quickly find meaningful patterns in external events. In fields that appeal to them, they have a fine power to organise a job and carry it through. Sceptical, critical, independent, determined, have high standards of competence and performance

INTP

Quiet and reserved. Especially enjoy theoretical or scientific pursuits. Like solving problems with logic and analysis. Interested mainly in ideas, with little liking for parties or small talk. Tend to have sharply defined interests. Need careers where some strong interest can be used and useful

ENFP

Warmly enthusiastic, high-spirited, ingenious, imaginative. Able to do almost anything that interests them. Quick with a solution for any difficulty and ready to help anyone with a problem. Often rely on their ability to improvise instead of preparing in advance. Can usually find compelling reasons for whatever they want

ENFJ

Responsive and responsible. Feel real concern for what others think or want, and try to handle things with due regard for others' feelings. Can present a proposal or lead a group discussion with ease and tact. Sociable, popular, sympathetic. Responsive to praise and criticism. Like to help others and enable people to achieve their potential

ENTP

Quick, ingenious, good at many things. Stimulating company, alert and outspoken. May argue for fun on either side of a question. Resourceful in solving new and challenging problems but may neglect routine assignments. Apt to turn to one new interest after another. Skilful in finding logical reasons for what they want

ENTJ

Frank, decisive, leaders in activities. Develop and implement comprehensive systems designed to solve organisational problems. Good in anything that requires reasoning and intelligent talk, such as public speaking. Are usually well informed and enjoy adding to their fund of knowledge

If you're still not sure which type best describes you, don't worry. It may help to go back to the descriptions of each dimension. Of course, the best way to identify your type is to complete the MBTI questionnaire and discuss your results with a trained and licensed practitioner.

Important points about MBTI type

Before we go on to apply your type to the issue of influencing, we'd like to stress a few important points about how you should use and view type.

➤ **You are more than your type.** Every person is unique. Your MBTI type is concerned with four important dimensions of difference in personality but it does not sum you up completely. For this reason, even if you compare yourself with someone of the same type, there will be many differences as well as similarities. Humans are far too complex to be summed up in four letters.

➤ **Type is about preferences, and is not a straitjacket**. We can still choose to act in ways different to our type. They are likely to consume more energy and concentration but, with practice, our performance will improve.

➤ **All types are equally valid**. There is no 'right' type. All have strengths and potential pitfalls. The aim is to use your insight to play to your strengths and make choices that will facilitate your growth and the development of others.

➤ **Type is an explanation, not an excuse**. Type provides useful insights into why we act in the way we do, but it cannot be used as an excuse for our actions.

Type and influencing

The most important lesson that type can teach us is that people are different. The MBTI describes differences in the way we are energised, the information we trust, the way we make decisions and the lifestyle we want. All these differences are valid and we should not fall into the trap of believing that our way is the only way. Even if you don't find MBTI theory helpful, we'd invite you to reflect on the sheer range of personalities who succeed in business or professional life. Some lead from the front, others influence from behind the scenes. Some put their success down to a grasp of detail, others keep their eye on the 'big picture'. Some rejoice in their readiness to ruthlessly hire and fire people according to their current usefulness, others treat their staff like extended family. And for every one who sees meticulous planning as essential, there's another who swears by bold, risk-taking ventures and seat-of-the-pants decision making. We must never assume that what works for us, works for everyone. Every personality type can be successful but each will be successful in a different way. And when it comes to influencing, each of us has to work out how we can succeed using our unique mix of personality, skills and experience.

Your default influencing style

Hopefully, you will have an idea by now of what your MBTI type might be. We're now going to use that type to think through how you tend to approach influencing people. This will give you some clues about your default influencing style – the approach you might naturally fall into. We realise that personality is not the only factor shaping our behaviour and there is an ongoing debate about the impact of personality as opposed to the influence of the situations we find ourselves in. But 'personality traits give rise to characteristic patterns of behaviour'[23] and therefore it is worth carefully considering what our MBTI type can tell us about how we tend to go about influencing people. For each preference, we've listed some of the things you might well naturally do as part of your influencing and some pointers for development.

Extraversion (E)	Introversion (I)
If you're an Extravert you might well...	If you're an Introvert you might well...
• develop extensive networks including in other departments	• prefer to network with a few, like-minded people
• be seen as outgoing and accessible	• be seen as reserved and private
• enjoy opportunities to meet new people	• enjoy developing existing contacts
• act before reflecting	• reflect before acting
• prefer face-to-face communication	• prefer written communication
• be happy to 'cold call'	• prefer to 'sell' to existing contacts
• be ready to speak off the cuff or take the lead in meetings	• let others speak unless you feel the need to do so
	• prefer to prepare before presenting your ideas
Pointers for developing as an influencer	Pointers for developing as an influencer
• Practise your listening skills	• Be more ready to speak out
• Practise reflection and thinking things through	• Be intentional about linking with people who can turn your ideas into action

Sensing (S)	Intuition (N)
If your preference is Sensing you might well...	If your preference is Intuition you might well...
• emphasise facts and current reality in your presentations and conversations	• emphasise future possibilities in your presentations and conversations
• prefer to discuss facts and figures: concrete data	• prefer to talk about trends and the 'big picture'
• like to be seen as practical and precise	• like to be seen as imaginative and creative
• see concrete data as persuasive	• see vision as persuasive
• see someone's experience and track record as persuasive	• see someone's potential and capacity for innovation as persuasive
• pay attention to the details of an issue but may miss the wood for the trees	• pay attention to the broad themes of an issue but may miss important details
Pointers for developing as an influencer	Pointers for developing as an influencer
• Practise being able to give a summarised overview of an issue rather than a detailed breakdown	• Make sure you have facts to back up your case
• Practise creative thinking	• Be able to demonstrate that you have thought through the practical implications of your proposal

Thinking (T)

If your preference is Thinking you might well...
- emphasise logic and objectivity in your presentations and conversations
- see logic as the trump card in any argument
- naturally point out flaws and weaknesses in others' positions
- be seen as impersonal and tough-minded
- upset or offend without knowing
- emphasise the 'right' answer
- enjoy robust debate and intellectual argument
- show helpfulness by addressing people's problems for them

Pointers for developing as an influencer
- Practise thinking through and be ready to talk about the human dimension of your proposal or idea. How will people benefit?
- Practise anticipating how others will feel about your decisions
- Practise expressing appreciation of others

Feeling (F)

If your preference is Feeling you might well...
- emphasise values and relationships in your presentations and conversations
- see human need or other deeply held values as more important than anything else
- naturally be appreciative and look for common ground
- be seen as 'tender hearted' and emotionally involved
- take issues too personally
- emphasise the impact on people
- enjoy creating harmony
- show helpfulness by empathising

Pointers for developing as an influencer
- Practise being able to present a logical basis for your proposal
- Remind yourself not to take all criticism personally. Treat it objectively and accept the bits that seem helpful
- Practise giving direct, objective feedback

Judging (J)

If your preference is Judging you might well...
- take a planned, structured approach to influencing
- focus on just those facts you consider relevant
- want closure, sometimes too soon
- be good at follow-through and doing what you say you will do
- prefer to stick to a plan, sometimes even when it is not going well
- find it hard to be flexible
- be seen as rigid or even controlling

Pointers for developing as an influencer
- Be ready to build in some flexibility to your plans for people who prefer it
- Consider whether you sometimes need to give people more space and time to think things through for themselves

Perceiving (P)

If your preference is perceiving you might well...
- seize opportunities as they arise, trust your ability to improvise
- look for a wide range of information
- keep options open, sometimes too long
- be enthusiastic and spontaneous
- be ready to change direction, particularly if it seems more interesting or exciting
- find it hard to stick to the plan, particularly if it involves routine or repetition
- be seen as indecisive or impetuous

Pointers for developing as an influencer
- Practise planning in advance your approach to an influencing issue ... then implementing the plan!
- Avoid taking on too much or spreading yourself too thinly

Doing what comes naturally

You can now begin to sketch out a picture of your probable influencing style and how people might see you. There are no 'wrong' types for influencing; each presents different strengths and potential pitfalls. Your default style is the one that goes 'with the grain' of your personality, the style you naturally adopt almost without thinking. And it is the 'without thinking' part that might cause problems, because if we can only influence in the way that suits our personality type, we are limiting our own effectiveness.

For example, imagine if Dave, an ENTP, needs to gain the support of several senior colleagues to introduce some new technology. Being an ENTP he prefers:

➤ face-to-face conversations (Extraversion)
➤ majoring on the exciting future potential the technology represents (Intuition)
➤ arguing his case robustly, stressing the objective logic of his argument (Thinking)
➤ seizing opportunities for conversations as and when they arise (Perceiving).

So, Dave has a succession of conversations which take place in corridors or after meetings where he enthusiastically outlines the benefits that the new technology will produce and strongly counters any arguments to the contrary. Despite his enthusiasm and energy, Dave is surprised that not all of his colleagues respond as favourably as he had hoped to what is obviously, to him at least, a great idea. He attributes this to not having made his case clearly enough and soon after is arriving unannounced in the offices of those not yet in agreement with him, or buttonholing them on their way to lunch to treat them to another, even more impassioned, informal presentation. When even this fails to win over the doubters, Dave is frustrated. He cannot see anything wrong with the way he has communicated his message. He can only conclude that his colleagues are being deliberately obstructive.

Does the story sound familiar? Perhaps you can identify with Dave as he goes about his task quickly and energetically. Or maybe, like some of his colleagues, you have been the focus of a well-intentioned but clumsy attempt to 'bring you on board'. Perhaps you have quietly observed this sort of thing happening around you and been able to see how misunderstandings arise and offence is taken. Personality type provides a way of understanding what is going on. Dave's influencing campaign was conducted according to how *he* likes to operate. He was doing what comes naturally. And for some people, it worked a treat. However:

➤ some of Dave's Introvert colleagues would have preferred to have time to think the idea through, or read about it, rather than just being buttonholed
➤ some of Dave's Sensing colleagues wanted to know the facts and figures, not just the big picture

➤ colleagues with a Feeling preference wanted to know what benefits for people
the new technology would bring and didn't enjoy having their questions just
batted aside

➤ colleagues with a Judging preference were put out by Dave arriving in their office
without an appointment or delaying them by stopping them in the corridor.

For some, Dave's approach was irritating. For others, he did not give them the type
of information they needed to make up their minds. Inevitably, this skewed their
view of his proposal. They were not being deliberately awkward, they were just
being human.

When Dave renewed his efforts by trying the same tactics again only more energetically, it was the equivalent of the tourist who thinks that if he speaks more and
more loudly, the locals will eventually understand him. Not only was he unlikely to
change anyone's mind, he also ran the risk of annoying them.

The cost of lack of self-awareness

In successful influencing we sometimes have to go beyond our natural preferences.
Otherwise we will only ever communicate with those who see the world as we do,
and there is a very real cost to this, as the following real-life example shows.

A very bright, highly articulate NHS Chief Executive came back from a course
at Harvard seized by the need to envision his staff. Unlike the bureaucratic stereo-
type, he was passionate about transforming his organisation into the finest possible provider of care. Like Dave in the fictional example above, he was an ENTP:
very outgoing and flamboyant, full of energy and with an impressive grasp of the
big issues of the day, he was a man of enthusiasms who was not always so good
at follow-through. He began to talk constantly about his vision for the future. He
used presentations, conversations, publications and training programmes to communicate his vision. Many responded well, catching his enthusiasm and the attractive picture of the future he presented. However, just as many were left cold by
his approach. While for him, getting the vision was an intuitive, almost religious
experience, others wanted a very practical explanation of why change was needed
and what it would mean for their day-to-day work. They were not energised by
vision, but by practical need. They were also annoyed by the way that, as it seemed
to them, one vision was swiftly followed by another. The Chief Executive's response
to these people was to see them as cynics or non-believers. Those who raised objec-
tions or asked too many questions were banished from the inner circle and passed
over when it came to promotion. This only heightened their dissatisfaction. The
irony was that it was the people who wanted to talk about the practicalities rather
than the big picture who were the ones the Chief Executive most needed. He was
increasingly surrounded by fellow visionaries who, like him, saw everyone else as

stuck-in-the-mud. But without practical, pragmatic people, his vision could never become reality. The people who could have turned big ideas into changes at ground level were treated badly and as a consequence became disaffected.

This failure of self-awareness, resulting in communication which reached only some of the staff, had a high cost. Instead of transformation there was frustration. Visionary initiatives quickly ran into the sand because of the lack of connection with day-to-day reality. A talented Chief Executive made only a fraction of the impact he could have achieved.

MBTI TYPES AND ORGANISATIONAL LEVEL

In research with a representative sample of the UK population,[24] it was found that at higher organisational levels there were significantly more NTJs (people with a preference for Intuition, Thinking and Judging) than non-NTJs. If this reflects a general trend, it would help explain top management's seeming preoccupation with logical analysis, long-term planning, innovation and the big picture at the possible expense of day-to-day practicality, people issues and flexibility. It may also explain why people with Sensing, Feeling or Perceiving preferences (and especially those with all three) might feel that their senior colleagues sometimes speak a different language.

Everyone has preferences when it comes to influencing. As an INFP, Andrew Price tends to prefer to work within his existing networks (Introversion) and to communicate mainly about strategy and change (Intuition). He majors on the development of people (Feeling) and has a spontaneous, unplanned approach to influencing (Perceiving). While there is nothing inherently wrong with these preferences, always staying within them can limit his effectiveness as an influencer. There are times when, for instance, a more planned approach which deliberately targets new people is needed or when a greater focus on detail and practicality would mean that more people are persuaded.

Giving people what they need – covering the bases

Knowing your personality type and your default influencing style is a good first step. What we then have to do is think through what people with other preferences might need. This will result in much more effective communication. We call this 'covering the bases', making sure that our influencing engages everybody, whatever their preference. The table opposite gives pointers you can use as you plan any form of influencing, from a single presentation to a long-term campaign. Use it as a checklist to quality assure your influencing approach. It is tempting to ignore or underplay the aspects we do not enjoy or which do not come naturally, but for some of our intended audience these factors are critical.

Giving people what they need – using the MBTI to improve your influencing

Their preference	Questions to ask yourself
Extraversion	• Are there opportunities to ask questions and interact? • Can people experience as well as hear about your key points through visits, role-play, etc.
Introversion	• Are there handouts and other reading material? • Will people have time to reflect and think things through?
Sensing	• Are supporting facts and figures available? • Are the implications for day-to-day work clear, now and in the future? If you are proposing changes, why are they needed and what practical problem will they solve? • What are the risks and have you addressed them?
Intuition	• How does your idea or proposal relate to the big issues of the day? • What are the opportunities and possibilities? • What is the underpinning model or concept?
Thinking	• Does your idea or proposal make logical sense? • Did you consider other options? • Can you demonstrate competence in this area?
Feeling	• How will people benefit? • Have you taken account of the values and feelings of individuals?
Judging	• Can you demonstrate that your approach is sufficiently well planned and organised? • Are timelines and deadlines clear?
Perceiving	• Is there room for manoeuvre within the overall plan? • Will you be flexible in the light of new facts or other people's contributions?

Asking these questions will help you to 'cover the bases' and avoid the trap of influencing in a way perfectly designed to only persuade people exactly like you!

Think for moment about the last time you tried to persuade a person or a group of people to take a certain course of action. This might have been a training session or a proposal to a management team. Reflect on the messages you gave and how you gave them.

➤ Did you cover the bases?

➤ Would people with MBTI preferences different from yours have found it easy to engage?

➤ What might you have done differently?

LEARNING ACTIVITIES

You'll get maximum value from this chapter if you take time to apply the main messages to the way you influence. Use the boxes below to write about and reflect on the issue of self-awareness.

GETTING FEEDBACK

Do you get good-quality feedback from your colleagues and your boss? If not, what could you do about this?

What messages have most stood out to you from feedback others have given you (whether you agreed with it or not!)?

PERSONALITY TYPE

Based on the descriptions in the chapter, what have you learned about your personality type?

What have you learned about your natural or default influencing style? What are the strengths and potential pitfalls of your style?

RECOMMENDED READING

If you want to pursue some of the ideas we touch on in this chapter, try the following books.

➤ For more on the MBTI: *Lifetypes* by Sandra Hirsh and Jean Kummerow (Warner Books). This book applies personality type to all areas of life, including work, learning and relationships.

➤ For more on emotional intelligence: *The New Leaders* by Daniel Goleman, Richard Boyatzis and Annie McKee (Sphere). Goleman and colleagues make the case that emotional intelligence is central to good leadership.

➤ For understanding what you are good at: *Now Discover Your Strengths* by Marcus Buckingham and Donald Clifton (Pocket Books). A very helpful book which includes a questionnaire to help you understand your strengths.

REFERENCES

1 Yukl G. *Leadership in Organisations*. Upper Saddle River: Prentice-Hall; 2002.
2 Fox S, Dewhurst F, Eyres J, Vickers D. *The Nature and Quality of Leadership in the Professions*. London: Council for Excellence in Management and Leadership; 2001.
3 Mintzberg H. *Managing*. Harlow: Prentice-Hall; 2009. p.9.
4 Palmer I, Hardy C. *Thinking about Management*. London: Sage; 2000.
5 Fullan M. *Leading in a Culture of Change*. San Francisco; Jossey-Bass; 2001. p.2.
6 Frohman D. *Leadership the Hard Way*. San Francisco: Jossey-Bass; 2008.
7 Tekleab AG, Sims HP Jr, Yun S, Tesluk PE, Cox J. Are we on the same page? Effects of self awareness of empowering and transformational leadership. *J Leadership Organiz Studies*. 2008; **14**(3): 185–201.
8 Young M, Dulewicz V. Relationships between emotional and congruent self-awareness and performance in the British Royal Navy. *J Manag Psychol*. 2007; **22**(5): 465–78.
9 Yammarino F, Attwater L. Do managers see themselves as others see them? Implications of self-other rating agreement for human resources management. *Organis Dynamics*. 1997; **25**(4): 35–44.
10 Ashford S, Tsui A. Self-regulation for managerial effectiveness: the role of active feedback seeking. *Acad Manage J*. 1991; **34**(2): 251–80.
11 Goleman D, Boyatzis R, McKee A. *The New Leaders*. London: Sphere; 2002.
12 Cranwell-Ward J, Bacon A, Mackie R. *Inspiring Leadership*. London: Thomson; 2002. p.78.
13 Barnard C. Mind in everyday affairs: an examination into logical and non-logical thought processes. *J Manage History*. 1995; **1**(4): 46–63.
14 Claxton G. *Hare Brain, Tortoise Mind: why intelligence increases when you think less*. London: Fourth Estate; 1997. p.211.
15 Price A. Weighting game. *Health Manage*. 2005; **Nov/Dec**: 24–6.
16 Greenleaf R. Tracing the past, present, and future of servant-leadership. In: Spears L, editor. *Focus on Leadership*. New York: Wiley; 2002. p.4.
17 Myers DG. *Intuition*. New Haven: Yale University Press; 2002.

18 West M, Patterson M. The workforce and productivity: people management is the key to closing the productivity gap. *New Economy*. 1999; **6**: 22–7.

19 West M. A matter of life and death. www.cihm.leeds.ac.uk/document_downloads/A_matter_of_life_and_death.pdf

20 Price A, Scowcroft A. *Essential Skills for Managing in Healthcare*. Oxford: Radcliffe; 2011.

21 Briggs Myers I with Myers P. *Gifts Differing*. Palo Alto: Consulting Psychologists Press; 1980.

22 Briggs Myers I. *Introduction to Type*. 6th ed. Oxford: Oxford Psychologists Press; 2000.

23 Hampson S. State of the art: personality. In: Henry J, editor. *Creative Management*. London: Sage; 1999.

24 Kendall E. *Myers–Briggs Type Indicator. Manual Supplement*. Oxford: Oxford Psychologists Press; 1998.

CHAPTER 3

Organisational culture

Just as people have different personalities, which affect how and why they act as they do, so do organisations. When people come together in the workplace they can adopt and display a collective set of behaviours that are often unique, or at least different from another group of people in the workplace next door.

The successful influencer learns how to spot those differences, demonstrates honour and respect for them, and then adopts approaches that will work well for each given situation. This chapter gives you the diagnostic tools, as well as the recommended responses, for dealing with the different ways in which organisations work.

In using the term 'organisation', we do not automatically mean the whole legal entity (medical facility, non-governmental organisation (NGO), health board, hospital, government body, etc.). The term applies equally to any work unit of more than one person and can therefore refer to a ward, work team, department, laboratory, office, clinic, division or directorate. The point here is that any collection of people working closely together will, over time, evolve a collective personality or character – some call it an ideology – and that, as with people, those identities are going to differ.

Why is this important? If you need to influence opinion and behaviour in an organisational setting you will not just be dealing with an individual's preferences and characteristics; you will have to take into account the organisational identity or ideology of where they work. The challenge is made that bit spicier by the fact that, just like people's personality preferences, the organisation's ideology is not written down anywhere. You cannot ask for a document or a website where the rules, rituals, conventions and subtle corrective methods are laid out in front of you. You have to spot the clues yourself, and then adapt your influencing behaviour so that you 'go with the grain' of that organisation. Just to add an extra layer of complexity to the topic, you may well find that many people working in a particular organisational unit will be blissfully unaware of the ideologies, or they will have no idea when and where they started. What you are likely to hear when you begin talking about the unique way each organisation goes about its business is 'That's the way it's always been done here'.

So far we have used a range of rather clumsy words to describe this organisational uniqueness – character, ideology, identity, personality. For both brevity and clarity, from now on we are going to use the word 'culture'. When we talk about an organisation's culture, we mean: *the unwritten rules, conventions, rituals and unspoken assumptions that guide internal and external behaviour, management processes (or the lack of them), and the way decisions are made and work challenges tackled.*

Let's make this personal and therefore memorable for you. Think back to the last time you made a significant job or career move. It may have been promotion within the same clinical or managerial specialty, a move between departments within the same health organisation, relocation to a different geographical area or even a complete change of profession and employment sector.

Now you have that experience clear in your mind, what did you notice that was different about the two workplaces?

Some of the changes would be quite obvious – new duties, new boss, working environment and layout, different IT systems, more/less money to spend, etc. These characteristics would be easy to spot and many of them would be in official documents or readily discussed inside and outside the team.

Think a bit harder now. There will have been other differences that were not written down, were rarely if ever discussed, and were often felt rather than seen. Here are some commonly reported examples to help prompt your thinking. The examples in each column do not come from the same organisation – they are merely illustrations of the contrasts in culture.

In one place...	In another...
We follow the hierarchy and refer strategic decisions upwards	If you want to know who makes the decisions around here, go and see 'Freda'
We are only interested in what you can offer this project	You need to have five years' experience at this level before this job comes your way
If X says yes, it's on!	The decision-making process is clear and well set out
We are about to implement this new procedure	We stopped doing that years ago
Is Fred in yet?	Has anyone seen Professor Biggins/the Director/ Dr Williams?
We need a senior representative from each discipline for this new working party	Let's get Jean, Linda and that new chap Bill to come up with some ideas
Let me know if things go wrong	Can we have a weekly/monthly update using the standard template?

None of the situations in this table is automatically right or wrong. However, each one is likely to have emerged as one of the ways in which that part of the organisation gets things done. It is only when we are used to one way and are then parachuted into that different world that the contrast becomes obvious.

In such situations it is easy, if not highly seductive, to instantly compare the new working environment with the one you have just come from and then judge that your new colleagues are either so much better or so much worse than those you have left. In this chapter we will suggest that what you are encountering is evidence of a different organisational culture. Not better, not worse, just different. Furthermore, we will strongly argue that unless and until you learn to identify these different cultures and then to honour and work with them, your attempts to influence colleagues who work outside your area will be seriously compromised. This is because it can be really hard to keep our preconceptions or judgements about how others go about their work private. When we let slip our puzzlement, amazement or sheer incredulity at others' behaviour, we lose credibility and gain an enemy.

THE DINNER GUEST FROM HELL!

Step back from the world of work for a moment and imagine that you have (perhaps foolishly) invited one of us for dinner at your house. At the appointed hour we duly arrive, bottle and/or flowers in hand, step into your house and say: '*Good grief, what possessed you to live in this area? Surely you could do better than this!*'.

Suppressing your desire to push me back out into the road, you would probably give a forced smile, deflect the question, get through the evening, and vow never again to allow this idiot into your house.

In this situation I have, with absolutely no authority or self-discipline, imposed my values and ideology (my culture) upon you, without stopping to consider that not only does your home and its location fit perfectly with you and your family, it is also *none of my business*. I have shown myself to be insensitive, intolerant, overbearing and superior. Now imagine that, during the meal, I wanted to introduce an idea for which I needed your help and support. Not surprisingly, my chances are about as warm as the dinner table atmosphere – sub-zero!

At one level this is merely a hypothetical domestic scenario. Yet in organisational settings, 'living choices' are being criticised daily, by people encountering colleagues in different departments and different cultures and then seeking to change them, to point out the errors of their ways, and to replace their ridiculous practices with shiny new ones. As a result, there are people working in those target organisations who have their backs put up on such a regular basis that they are, quite reasonably, refusing to have anything to do with the other person and their ideas. The person with the ideas returns to their own work area empty-handed, thinking 'What's wrong with these people, do they behave like this deliberately, do they care about what we are trying to do?', etc., etc.

As we covered in Chapter 1, once we have decided that *'it's their fault'* it lets us off the hook and we can sit there content in our total rightness.

The simple fact is that different organisational groups have evolved their own culture because that is what works for them. The evolution may have been driven by the nature of the tasks they undertake, the risks and rewards of success and failure, or as a way of managing external expectations. It may have been the vision and passion of a single driving figure or the conventions and rules of the leading profession with that department. Conversely, that culture may have arisen in response to a rapidly changing external environment and the need to respond flexibly and rapidly. You need to accept a simple but perhaps uncomfortable truth.

> If the people working in that 'other' culture can either assist with or hold back progress on your ideas and plans, you need to start by acknowledging their right to be different, and then adapt your influencing style to work with the grain of that culture rather than against it.

To take any other approach is to guarantee failure. After all, if you were on the receiving end of someone else's influencing and they either failed to honour your internal culture or actively criticised it, how much time would you give to their idea? In addition, the next time they came into view, how open would you be to their overtures?

It seems that in the world of influencing the guiding phrase should not be: *Do as you would be done by,* but: *Do as* <u>they</u> *would be done by*!

For the remainder of this chapter we are going to outline for you a framework of organisational culture that you can then use to spot and understand the cultures around you. Not only will the model give you valuable clues and insight as to why the different cultures behave as they do, we will also provide you with tried and tested influencing strategies that work with each one. You need to acknowledge that many of these strategies are bespoke; in other words, they are not interchangeable across several cultures, and you will see why as we discuss the different types.

We should straight away acknowledge a huge debt to two writers who have not only developed and then refined this model, but have unwittingly left enough space for future writers like us to customise it for an environment such as healthcare.

Roger Harrison is credited with developing the original model, in which he identified four organisational ideologies. His article *Understanding your organisation's character*[1] argued that many of the tensions within organisations were caused by clashes between these ideologies. By way of context, Harrison described an organisation's ideology as:

The systems of thought affecting the behaviour of its people, its ability to meet their needs and demands, and the way it copes with its external environment. (p.119)

Harrison's four ideologies, which we will now call cultures, were as follows (the synopses in brackets are our summaries of Harrison's explanations).

➤ **Power orientation** (Power is good and is used to gain internal compliance and to repel external threat)

➤ **Role orientation** (Rationality and order are good, and offer legality, legitimacy and responsibility)

➤ **Task orientation** (Goal achievement is good and matters more than process, authority and structure)

➤ **Person orientation** (Meeting the personal needs of the members is good and nothing else should compromise this objective)

Harrison argued that the norms, behaviours, assumptions and unwritten rules in a particular work area all combined to produce and protect a particular culture, and he went on to assess how well equipped each cultural type was to meet six important interests, three of which were personal and three of which were organisational.

1 Interests of people
   ➤ Security against economic, political or psychological deprivation
   ➤ Opportunities to voluntarily commit to meaningful goals
   ➤ The pursuit of growth and self-development

2 Organisational interests
   ➤ Effective response to threat and danger
   ➤ Rapid and flexible response to change
   ➤ Internal integration and management

As we explore the four cultures introduced by Harrison in 1972, you will be able to make up your own mind as to how each culture might perform in protecting those interests. However, the main reason for discussing the model here is its usefulness in developing influencing strategies.

The second writer is Charles Handy, whose further development of Harrison's model has made it so accessible today. Well known in the UK and abroad, Handy has an enviable reputation for explaining the complex world of organisations and management with both clarity and simplicity. In his book *Understanding Organisations*, originally published in 1985, Handy made the connection between the four cultures – power, role, task and person – and the characteristics of mythical Greek gods. Indeed, Handy subsequently published a whole book on this subject, entitled appropriately *Gods of Management*.[2]

At first glance, you might think that Handy has taken a perfectly valid model, if somewhat dry and sober, and trivialised it by introducing a bunch of made-up deities from Mount Olympus. However, he succeeded in making the cultures instantly recognisable and easily remembered. He also offered a series of images (one for each culture) that, in themselves, gave further clues and reinforcements as to how and why the different cultures behave as they do. This 'perfect storm' of 1970s social psychology, Handy's characterisation of Greek gods, and the simple yet powerful imagery for each culture have given us a rare gift – a model of organisational thinking that is both immediately accessible and instantly useful.

As we run through each of the four cultures, their associated gods and the images, we would invite you to do two things.

First, please acknowledge, as we do, that no organisation is going to be a perfect fit with just one culture, with no traces of the others within it.

Second, begin to evaluate your own work team and those around you as you learn about the four cultures. In other words, make the model relevant straight away. You may find that it is easier to spot the culture of others than of your own work area and this is quite common. Some years ago, one of us coined the phrase 'a fish does not know what it is to be wet', meaning that if we have only ever known the way things are done around here, we may struggle to even find words to describe it. However, as your cultural antennae are tuned in you will become more adept at spotting the clues all around you.

ZEUS

The first of the four cultures is Harrison's **power** culture. Handy associated this with the Greek god Zeus. Hardly surprising really. Zeus was god of gods, the all-powerful and he had the power to make or break the other gods. All power remained with him and only close allies were given the slightest room for manoeuvre and local autonomy. The image that Handy chose to allocate to this Zeus culture is the spider's web.

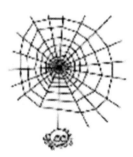

In a Zeus culture, there will be a central power figure, like a spider connected to the centre of their web. The radials in the web signify that Zeus ensures that everything and everyone is connected to them. The Zeus figure, who could be male or female, is often also the most senior person in the formal structure, but not always. We have encountered primary care practices where the senior partner is senior in title only. The real power (never openly acknowledged, of course) is held elsewhere, having been cultivated by a series of alliances, deals, naked power or even marriage. In some practices where the practice manager is also the spouse of the senior partner, it is quite easy to see that the real power might be 'behind the throne' rather than on it! The spider's web diagram also helps us to understand that different people have different amounts of delegated power, dependent on how close to the centre they are. We have come across organisations where some of the most senior people (at least by their title) have virtually no influence at all when it comes to the big decisions and, if they were to be placed on the spider's web, it would be at the margins at best. Conversely, there are those whose job role and title suggest that they are relatively junior yet they are at the heart of everything. On our spider's web they would be close to the centre, literally in the 'inner circle'.

So far we have revealed the Zeus culture as having an all-powerful central figure, surrounded by an inner circle of confidants whose presence at the top table sometimes belies their lowly official status. Power is absolute, and Zeus has the power to either make or break the lives and careers of those around him or her.

Here are some of the other clues that might suggest you are dealing with a Zeus culture.

Internal relationships

Progress is by patronage and is a highly fragile affair. A rise to prominence is more likely to be the result of pleasing Zeus than via any planned methodical career progression but, given the volatile nature of Zeus' benevolence, such favours are as easily lost as they are won. People can be flavour of the month one day and an outcast the next, sometimes without even knowing why either 'honour' was bestowed upon them.

Force will be met with force, whether the Zeus character became so powerful through deliberate or accidental means. This does not imply that all Zeus characters are corrupt or obsessed with power for its own sake. Many Zeus cultures we have encountered are led by quite charismatic and benevolent characters who genuinely believe that what they offer is focus, clarity, passion, and drive. In such circumstances they may interpret a challenge to their authority as risking a drop in performance or reputation. Their desire to keep power is then easily explained as 'staying true to what we are trying to do here', not a malicious greed for power.

Staff in Zeus organisations will devote much of their time to anticipating and second-guessing what Zeus wants or how he or she might respond to their actions and decisions. This can lead to a culture of 'upward delegation' whereby it is safer, and less noisy, to escalate decisions along the radials of the spider's web so that those close to Zeus make the final decisions. Even when access to Zeus is not possible, you may find staff making their decisions on the basis of 'would Zeus approve if and when they found out?'. They will often make their decision on the basis of precedent rather than the unique circumstances of the presenting problem. It seems that, if this is what Zeus decided last time, we will do the same again now.

It is not uncommon to hear two types of argument going on in a Zeus culture. The first will be short and top down, and will normally involve Zeus admonishing someone who has incurred his or her wrath. The second will be more extended and will be between Zeus and someone who has earned the right to be trusted. In such scenarios, everyone still knows that Zeus will make the final decision but the central figure quite enjoys intellectual sport with the more feisty members of their inner circle. Do not be fooled by these arguments. The markings on the pitch are quite clear and the final decision will be Zeus'. The moment that Zeus feels truly threatened by one of their followers, that person would quickly find themselves on the margins of the spider's web, with little or no influence. Their job title and pay will remain the same, but they will be neutralised.

Fad and whim

Zeus figures tend to be totally focused on one issue or idea for a while but then completely taken with a new approach, at which point the whole organisation has to divert its resources to the new venture. This apparent self-indulgence, treating the organisation almost as a plaything, is often subconscious and Zeus characters rarely appreciate the impact on their workforce. If they do find out, it is likely that some brave and trusted lieutenant has finally whispered in Zeus' ear and lived to tell the tale.

Communications

Meetings and other communications in this culture tend to be short, loud and one-way. Paper is often seen as unhelpful or a distraction and may be given little priority. Absolute compliance is expected and any alternatives to Zeus' own ideas will need to be truly spectacular, as well as non-threatening, to get any airtime.

Risks

One of the inherent risks with Zeus culture is that there will almost certainly be one or more blind spots. If Zeus refuses to, or cannot, see a problem or opportunity, there is little chance of the rest of the organisation being rewarded for spending any time on it. The focus and drive that so often are Zeus' most valuable attributes can easily become, to continue the mythology, their Achilles heel.

A now retired senior (Zeus) manager once said to one of us: 'Our general practitioners will never really take on minor surgery ... so we will continue to build our hospital-based minor surgery unit'. All attempts to show that this was a false assumption were met with stubborn refusal and, in some cases, the critics were transferred out of the team. Soon the whole organisation accepted Zeus' version of events and little time was spent on planning for an alternative scenario. As predicted by those dissenting voices in the team, GP fundholding was introduced in the UK shortly afterwards and many local GPs quickly developed their own minor surgery capability. Funding was diverted to primary care and the new unit was underused until its eventual closure.

Zeus as an instrument of change

As you read this aggregated account of the Zeus culture, two thoughts may have struck you. The first is that Zeus is mentioned a lot in the narrative. This is both true and relevant, because that central figure has their fingerprints on virtually everything that goes on, either directly or due to staff ensuring that things go the way Zeus wants. The second thought is that we might have painted quite a negative, almost pathetic, picture of Zeus and their culture. If so, let us correct that now.

Zeus cultures are genuinely exciting places to work, principally because things get done quickly, with little fuss, no procrastination and scant regard for pomp or ceremony. As a result, *if* the things getting done are the things you would like done, you are likely to see Zeus as 'a breath of fresh air', 'just what we need' and 'a kick up the pants for the system'. As a result, Zeus characters are often in demand by politicians when parts of their domain are in need of a jump-start.

In the 1980s the Conservative UK government sought to bring a more results-orientated dynamism to the healthcare system, signalling a move away from a consensus style of management that was seen as slow and lethargic. As a result, a number of senior figures from the world of business, enterprise and the military were drafted in, given the title general manager and actively encouraged to shake things up a bit. Many of these incoming executives found that whilst they had been asked to be decisive and dynamic, the rest of the healthcare infrastructure was unprepared for this and reacted accordingly. Within a few years most of the new cohort had either retired or returned to their previous sectors, complaining of an inability to turn their decisions into sustainable action on the ground and lack of political support from above when things became turbulent and confrontational, particularly with the large and powerful professions.

Even in the 21st century, there is evidence that if and when a hospital is deemed to be failing, local and national politicians still favour bringing in the turnaround specialist who cuts through the deadwood, makes things happen, and is less concerned with the ruffled feathers. Many of them succeed, but some find themselves in the same position as their 1980s counterparts, pulling on the levers of power in their office only to find that, due to the sheer complexity of healthcare organisations, there is nothing connected to those levers.

In contrast, if Zeus figures divert their time and effort into matters that do not meet with your approval you are more likely to judge them as obstinate, bullying, self-centred and unwilling to listen.

Alas, it seems that Machiavelli was right in that:

> It ought to be remembered that there is nothing more difficult to take in hand, more perilous to conduct, or more uncertain in its success, than to take the lead in the introduction of a new order of things. Because the innovator has for enemies all those who have done well under the old conditions ... [3]

History has given us a rich source of Zeus cultures to reflect upon. In the world of business, there is little doubt that the publishing mogul Robert Maxwell operated a Zeus culture. In politics, UK Prime Ministers Thatcher and Blair have certainly been written about by those who know them well in ways that suggest Zeus tendencies. Intriguingly, more recent political events in the UK suggest that it may have been Lord Mandelson rather than Prime Minister Gordon Brown who was the Zeus figure in the last Labour Cabinet (2007–10). If correct, this would be a good example of the Zeus power being located in a different place from that implied by the organisational chart.

Closer to our healthcare home, we know of several senior executives and medical figures who have not only operated a Zeus culture but have appeared to actively cultivate that image. One in particular seemed to delight in his staff never quite knowing whether today was a good day or a bad day to enter the office, and another has made a successful career being brought into hospitals where managerial/medical relations have been poor and introducing a strong dose of corrective medicine.

An ex head of a civil service health department had an undisguised poor opinion of the managers in their area and wasted few opportunities to state that opinion in public places and conferences. Whilst this gained considerable support from those professions who had endured the actions of said managers, the culture of fear and hesitation it generated led, ironically, to high turnover and even worse performance in the future.

Finally, many a medical student will argue that their experience of medical teams is such that, whilst in theory it is a highly structured affair with junior, senior, specialist and consultant grades, they regularly came across consultants who ran the entity as a Zeus culture.

So, there you have the Zeus culture, complete with all its idiosyncrasies, its attractive strengths and its potential for self-inflicted wounds. As we said at the start of this section, you are unlikely to come across a work unit where this is the *only* visible culture, but it is often the dominant one in smaller pockets of larger organisations. Where it does manifest itself at the top of a large workplace, it has immense capacity for making positive change happen quickly. However, on rare occasions, it can also leave a legacy of hurt and stifled innovation.

If your reflection suggests that this is the culture you have to get alongside and influence, then we will offer you some approaches that will work later in this chapter. However, before you leap straight to the answers, we invite you to learn about the other three cultures first as it may be that your initial diagnosis changes once you have more information about the alternatives.

APOLLO

Our second cultural type is the one Harrison calls the **role** culture. You will recall that this culture promotes rationality and order, both in its work and in its structure, believing that such an approach gives it legitimacy and authority. Handy has chosen the Greek god Apollo to help describe this culture and has also offered the image of a stone temple to show some of its characteristics.

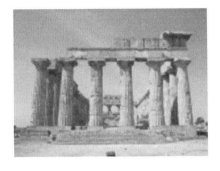

Handy's combination of mythical god and image is significant. In mythology, Apollo was (amongst other attributes) the god of order and rules. The temple image is a perfect match for this culture due to its firm base, strong individual columns or pillars and a triangle at the top that spans all of the supporting structure. If you have one close to hand, take out a copy of your organisation's management structure diagram. The similarity between typical structure charts and the Apollo temple image will be striking, as the former will show a top management team (the triangle), a series of functional departments or specialisms (the pillars) and a solid base of junior workers and systems (the base).

Another way to think about the Apollo culture is that it is the culture of bureaucracy. We need to stress that, when we use that term, we are merely describing a way of organising work. Of course, the term is often used in a judgemental and pejorative sense, as in 'bureaucracy gone mad' or ' the dead hand of bureaucracy', but in this book we offer the word free of any value judgements.

Let's move on to some of the assumptions and behaviours suggesting that the people you need to influence are working in an Apollo role culture.

Process orientation

This culture is primarily concerned with process and procedure (remember that Apollo the god preferred order and rules). The mindset is that these procedures and rules protect quality and reduce the risk of variance or mistakes. Apollo is almost always a risk-averse culture, much to the irritation of Zeus cultures who see those people as unambitious, plodding and timid. You will often find that this culture would prefer not to make a decision rather than risk making a bad decision, but as an outsider you need to understand that this is a well-developed and successful strategy, not a deliberate attempt to ruin your day!

Respect and deference

As Harrison's original label of the Role culture implies, there is more weight and respect given to the role or job title people have than the person actually doing that job. For this reason, there is a precision and wordiness to job titles not seen in other cultures. It is not uncommon to see job roles with titles like Deputy Directorate Manager, ENT, Maxillo-Facial and Oncology (West Sector), and the post holder will be subtly encouraged to rejoice in that status rather than apologise for its word count. The post holder is not unimportant, just less so than the status attached to the post, and the Apollo culture will often bestow considerable respect and deference on a senior post, even if there is a general view around the office that the post holder is quite poor at their job.

An interesting manifestation of this role deference is that people will often be addressed, particularly in meetings and official documents, by their job title or even the initials of their job title, rather than by name. It seems that this formality is both normal and expected, even if the people involved know each other well and use first names freely around the office.

> Some years ago one of us attended a policy meeting involving senior civil servants and health professionals, held in a government building. It was a closed meeting but with a highly structured agenda and chairing style. All the members worked closely with each other but we were startled when the Chairman turned to Jean (not her real name), his Chief Nursing Officer colleague, to lead the next topic, and said 'CNO, would you introduce item 7 please?'. This default style of using official titles is unique to Apollo and is therefore an immediate clue as to how you are expected to behave in your dealings with the culture.

Apollo organisations are extremely hierarchical and they attach great importance to pay and relative grading differentials, as they demonstrate the floors and ceilings of responsibility for each job in the structure. There will often be detailed and elaborate explanations of levels of responsibility. Some of these relate to authority to hire staff, degrees of disciplinary action that can be taken per grade level, and financial expenditure limits. It is common to find that, as you rise through the career ranks, the amount you can spend on a single purchase without higher approval also increases, but to the outsider the levels seem both low and arbitrary. The key to understanding these rigid procedures is that they are there to reduce risk (see above). In many public sector bureaucracies, they also serve to demonstrate safe stewardship of public funds, even if the transaction costs of maintaining the audit trail may be more expensive than any inappropriate expenditure caused by having no checks and balances.

Progression and communication

As already hinted, career progression in Apollo is normally vertical and hierarchical, with great care taken to define job descriptions and role profiles, followed by carefully orchestrated recruitment and interview processes. Demonstrating competence and soundness is rewarded and the recruitment process tends to screen out serial risk takers and mavericks. There is often an unintended hypocrisy at work in Apollo organisations in that innovation and creativity are sought (in response to political and public clamour for a more dynamic management style) but those making appointment decisions may be unsettled by the risk involved and end up appointing safer candidates who can demonstrate 'appropriate experience for the post'.

Added to this hierarchical career progression, communication is often along clearly defined lines (normally up and down the functional pillars). Cross-pillar communications are not actively discouraged but the structure does not always make them easy to achieve, with the result that such organisations are often criticised for their silo working or bunker mentality. Progressive governments around the world have been extolling the virtues of joined-up working in their respective public sectors for many years now but the well-worn pathways of communication – up the pillars, across the top and then down the next pillar – make that integrated working much harder to achieve. Some have made progress and have redrawn their organisation charts to show a closer connection between, say, health and local government social care services. However, the mere act of producing another organisational chart risks solidifying these new communications channels into a new Apollo culture.

Evidence is king

In keeping with Apollo's desire for order and stability, it is a very data-hungry culture, valuing evidence, analysis, options, calm consideration, consultation, policy integration, etc., all words that outsiders see as really meaning 'action avoidance'. This can be quite unfair on occasion because all Apollo is trying to do is make sure that the decisions made are right, sustainable and appropriate within the broader context in which they operate. Apollo hates rushed decisions, as they are often seen as wrong or ill thought through. As you place Zeus and Apollo side by side you can immediately see the battle lines being drawn!

In order to manage this somewhat reflective and inclusive process of decision making, Apollo is likely to be underpinned by committees, meetings, paper, project groups, etc., all of which tend to add to the time taken to move from issue to action. Some consultation processes have a statutory process and timescale but even where this is not the case, Apollo will see timescales measured in months or years as perfectly normal and even necessary to ensure that the eventual action is defensible.

Option appraisal is a key tool for Apollo and is often a key reason why other cultures fail to make headway in their negotiations with Apollo staff. You should bear in mind that soundness and integrity are core values for Apollo, they need reassurance that the proposals put to them stand on their own merits and are free of any 'personal benefits' to the person making the proposal. Other cultures tend to rush in and demand that their project is approved. Even though they may have undertaken some review of the alternatives within their own organisation, they fail to include this analysis in their proposal, leaving Apollo uneasy. This culture needs answers to these sorts of questions.

➤ Where is the evidence that we need to change at all?

➤ Of course, *you* want this project to proceed – you will benefit – but where are the independently assessed alternatives?

➤ Do you have independent support?

➤ What are the potential knock-on effects for other parts of our policy in this area?

➤ Might saying yes set an unhelpful precedent?

Other cultures can easily see these as avoiding tactics, become frustrated as a result, and once again the conflict lines are drawn. We are certainly not excusing 'job's worth' behaviours in any culture and we do not believe that every Apollo culture has perfect motives. However, as a general rule, this culture wants to get it right, maximise the sustainability of its work, and minimise the downside. To do this, they are often prepared to have no decision rather than a bad one!

Process, procedure and protocol are highly prized in Apollo cultures, even if some of its own staff tend to complain about the amount of red tape. It is important to acknowledge why having a procedure for everything is so important in these organisations. Apollo bureaucracies are often very good at what we call repeatability. In other words, they put in place a level of service or performance and then use their protocols to maintain that level day in, day out until the need for change is overwhelming.

It works!

Everyone reading this book benefits in some way from this Apollonian obsession with procedure, even though we often like to disparage both the protocols and those enforcing them. Unless you work for yourself, your wage/salary is calculated by an Apollo culture. Your expenses claims are managed in the same way. The fact that, for the most part, you can rely on and make future decisions based on a stable level of remuneration is down to Apollo. If you had a car accident, your insurance company would use a standardised, 'fair' assessment process to calculate blame and compensation. Law making and enforcement run along Apollo lines. In healthcare, care pathways, medication dispensing, theatre instrument management, laboratory testing, etc. all rely on a standardised protocol and lives could be at risk if there was any variation. Imagine managing any of these process-driven tasks using the spontaneity, volatility and emotions associated with Zeus. As a patient in hospital, would you like your medication administered by Apollo or by someone who has decided on a whim that 'today we are all taking pink ones'?

Pervasive and resilient

As we have been setting out the character of Apollo cultures (hopefully avoiding too much mischievous stereotyping), you will see that Apollo is all around us.

National and local government departments, the Civil Service, many work units inside healthcare organisations, even the Catholic Church, they are all examples of Apollo. TV viewers in the UK will no doubt remember the political satire/comedy programme *Yes Minister*, with its ongoing duel between the Minister and his Permanent Secretary, Sir Humphrey Appleby, a figure who clearly relished everything Apollo! His ability to take the Minster's desire for action and headlines and quietly bog them down in the machinations of the Civil Service has brought a wry smile to the lips of many politicians and commentators.

All Apollo cultures are remarkably resilient and long lasting, principally because they offer a largely safe and efficient way of delivering core tasks with consistency and low risk. Just like the Greek temple image that Handy associates with this culture, they can withstand great upheaval and turbulence. Indeed, if you take the temple metaphor a little further, you will see that even earthquakes fail to topple the pillars or destroy the base, although most temple ruins have lost their top structure!

This suggests that whilst top managers and clinical specialists may come and go (leaders being easy to remove in the wake of 'seismic' events such as scandals, enquiries and political demands), the day-to-day work of most Apollo organisations will carry on largely unchanged. A sobering thought for those who have reached the top of their Apollonian careers!

In the world of healthcare, you will often encounter Apollo cultures within many corporate functions such as finance, payroll, HR, audit, PR and the business of managing the legal Board processes. We believe that many clinical professions also operate under Apollo principles. Nursing, therapies, science-based professions, etc. often have quite rigid structures, with strict job titles, competence thresholds, grade labels, colour-coded uniforms, and a heavy reliance on protocols and pathways. In the UK in particular, these professions have moved from pay grading structures based on words through ones based on letters of the alphabet, to the current system using the numbers 1 to 8. It is quite common to hear senior staff and even the professionals themselves refer to colleagues by their 'band number'. We even know of one organisation whose Band 6 staff regularly attend a meeting which is itself entitled 'the Band 6 meeting'. At one level all this is merely shorthand designed to give clarity and brevity to any conversation. However, we suspect that it reveals a deeper, unspoken set of Apollo assumptions and values that the job has primacy, not the person doing it.

So, to summarise Apollo, it is a risk-averse, process-driven culture where consistency and order are valued as ways of achieving repeatable results. It will be present in some parts of virtually every organisation of any size, where getting things organised and being methodical are valued.

As with Zeus, Apollo is capable of both great deeds and miserable performance.

Apollo will keep your activities legal, will keep its leaders out of jail, will make sense of chaos and complexity and will ensure your organisation lives long and prospers.

At times it will drive those around it to distraction with its apparent obsession with process over outcome. This slowness to change, which those within it prize as being the best defence against error, means that it can easily be overtaken by events or fail to capitalise on fleeting opportunities. Apollo organisations are notoriously vulnerable to gradually deteriorating external conditions and may not spot the dangers until it is too late. Examples of this include the challenges of maintaining service provision in the face of an ageing population, and preventing the deterioration of care quality that can result in scandals and serious failures in care. In the former, healthcare organisations have known for years that an ageing population will reduce the size of the workforce pool and increase the demands placed on clinical services. There is plenty of thought and consideration going on but some commentators believe that, by the time the service acts, it will be too little, too late. Similarly, enquiry after enquiry into the abuse and deaths caused by failures in care seem to ask the same question.

> We have been here before and were told lessons would be learned last time, but here we are again. Why does this keep happening?

Given Apollo's predilection for process, it is often the case that their response to such enquiries is a public commitment to remove one or more of the top managers and 'review our procedures'. Whilst this is often right and proper, as a way of engaging with inflamed public opinion it can sound somewhat inadequate and may be seen as more evidence that the problem is not being taken seriously.

SELF-REFLECTION 2

Before we move on to the third cultural type, we invite you once again to pause and look around you. Where are the Apollo cultures in your world? Are you in one or do you perhaps have regular dealings with colleagues who operate an Apollo culture? Reflect on the way negotiations and influencing activities have gone in the past. Was there a genuine attempt to understand and then work with the differences in approach or was there more 'criticising' going on? If you are not sure whether the organisation you are trying to deal with is Apollo, what might you do to find out?

Make your own notes here.

ATHENA

Our third cultural type was originally described by Harrison as the **task** culture. Earlier we summarised this as a place where getting the job done was seen as more important than how things were organised, and here we give you more information and clues to help you spot this culture at work. Handy linked the task culture with the goddess Athena. As with many mythical gods, Athena was associated with a wide range of abilities and interests, but the ones we are interested in here are her associations with *war, crafts and skills*, for reasons that will become apparent in a moment. The image chosen by Handy to reinforce the characteristics of Athena cultures is a grid or matrix. Again the reasons will emerge from the following description.

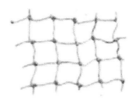

In a typical Athena culture, there are three Ts at work.
➤ **Task:** the job to be done
➤ **Team:** the right mix of skills for the task
➤ **Trust:** the team is left to manage the task as they see fit

Many people say they would prefer to work in an Athena culture, due to its emphasis on self-management, freedom and creativity. It seems to resonate with a 21st-century view of organisational life and the decline of paternalistic management regimes. Paradoxically, it is the culture that many organisations fail to get right, principally because the 'letting go' required by senior managers is OK in theory but difficult to deliver in practice. You will see why as we go through the description.

Devolution

The prevailing belief system in an Athena culture is that the team on the ground is best placed to know what is required, will deliver if left to get on with it, and that talent is more important than status. For this reason the culture is often associated with the terms 'devolved management' and 'self-managed teams'.

In contrast to Apollo, the Athena culture strives to ensure that the make-up of the team is based purely on the task to be addressed or the work to be delivered. Skills and track record are more highly prized than status or hierarchy and it is common for teams to be handpicked for the job.

Fluidity

One of the signs that you may be encountering an Athena culture is that people will often be part of several work teams at the same time. Because the hierarchy is less important, people are invited to work in several areas, based purely on the relevance of their skills to the task at hand. For this reason, project teams are the weapon of choice in Athena, with the teams forming, reforming, disbanding and changing membership as and when new projects arise. This fluidity makes drawing an accurate and relevant organisational chart difficult but typical Athenians seem not to care. Everyone knows who their boss is, but that person may not be the colleague they report to on a daily basis for the project(s) they are working on. Indeed, it is possible that their formal line manager will be on a project team that their subordinate is leading.

The grid or matrix image offered by Handy takes some explaining but you will see its relevance. If you see the intersections in the grid as the local work areas or problems, then the lines act as supply routes for things like the funding, the equipment, the information and the authority to act. In other words the corporate organisation is there to support and feed the local work teams, not vice versa. Whilst neither Harrison nor Handy gives this example, we think the analogy of special forces such as the British SAS offers a good example of Athena.

> Imagine that there is unrest in a far-flung part of the empire. Intelligence suggests that a small team of experts should be sent to sort things out. Based on analysis of the problem, the right mix of skills (weapons, communications, interpreter, logistics and jungle warfare) is selected. The new team is then sent over the border with authority to act as they see fit and then left alone to get on with the job. Finally the team is extracted from the area when the problem is solved and then that team disbands only for the members to join new teams as new problems emerge.

In most organisational settings the work teams are likely to be more stable and long term but the central principles remain.

➤ Involvement is based on technical contribution.
➤ The operating parameters are set by the corporate organisation.
➤ The team is equipped for the job.
➤ The team is then allowed considerable latitude to make things happen.

If you are wondering what this has to do with the healthcare sector, then think about the clinical directorate model. In theory, it is based purely on Athena principles. There is a belief that devolved management is better than remote command

and control, the local team is given the budget and freedom to act, and the work unit is based around specific clinical areas. A joint working approach is encouraged by clustering all the different professions around the common aim of improving patient care. Some corporate health departments such as estates, information management and technology (IMT), and HR often operate along similar lines, with staff assigned to projects or work areas rather than simply offering a 'one size fits all' service.

Challenge and motivation

One of the factors that encourage an Athena culture is the setting of problems and challenges. Typically, Athenians want to tackle things, preferably new things, and often report that pitting their wits against the issue is highly motivational. Athena is less interested in maintenance and routine, due to the perception that there will be insufficient challenge to keep them sharp.

In the field of healthcare, the theory of Athena is not always borne out in reality. The principal reason for this is the power of Apollo. Indeed, many of the healthcare organisations we have worked with over the years display a clear schizophrenia and constant struggle between the freedoms sought by devolved teams and the desire for the corporate entity to keep control and minimise risk. It seems that even in the 21st century devolution is seen as risky. As a consequence, many clinicians who were encouraged into clinical director posts report that the 'promised' freedom to act locally was either absent or severely curtailed. At the beginning of this chapter we quoted an occasion where a chief executive exhorted the troops to innovate, challenge and make things happen (Athena). He was swiftly followed by a lieutenant requesting business plans submitted in standard form (Apollo). This disconnect between theory and practice is a regular source of tension between clinicians and corporate managers, even where the latter have had extensive careers in clinical fields. This serves to emphasise just how pervasive organisational culture can be, despite the wishes and skills of the staff concerned.

Other examples of Athena would be advertising agencies (who put together a team to meet the client's brief and disband that team once the contract is fulfilled) and consultancy firms.

The implications of being Athena

On the surface Athena sounds good and many readers will see it as preferable to the stereotypical self-indulgence of a Zeus culture and the perceived bureaucracy of Apollo. Indeed, anecdotal experience suggests that, properly run and supported, Athena organisations are exciting and creative places to work. However, there are prices to be paid by all involved for this outcome to be achieved.

➤ The first is that the organisation is still responsible for setting the overall direction of the entity and issuing any non-negotiables within which the work teams need to operate (and the devolved teams need to accept this). We call these non-negotiables the 'markings on the pitch', the things which make clear what game is being played, what the rules are and what shape ball is being used. With these rules in place, the sports team is free to be as creative as they wish, in support of that overall goal.

➤ Second, the senior staff must be prepared to step back and not micro-manage. As we just suggested, this is very difficult if Athena sits within a broader Apollo environment, and even more tricky when there is a political dimension at the top (e.g. the public sector in the UK). A colleague described an ideal managerial approach for Athena: 'hands on, fingers out'. The first part of this conveys interest, support and open communication; the second part reminds us of the need to let the teams do things their way and be prepared to have them come up with different approaches to our own. One of the most damaging things you can do to Athena is to say you trust them but then spend the rest of the time asking for reports, updates, proposals and approval forms.

➤ Third, and most worrying, you may have to accept that Athena organisations will not always be the most efficient. There are two reasons for this. One is that the teams can be so focused on their own problem or sector that opportunities for joint working and integration can easily be lost. Some teams seem to actively work against the interests of another, leading to one team solving a problem only for this to create a new problem elsewhere in the system. The other reason for any inefficiency is that the corporate services, finance, IT, HR, planning, etc., may be overstretched supporting so many devolved work teams. A common solution to this is for each team to have its own finance or HR person, and this may lead to corporate overheads being higher than if Apollo was running things.

As long as the overall management regime accept this change of role from controlling to supporting, and commit their energies to connecting the work of the disparate work teams, Athena can be a powerful force for change. Conversely, if the organisation carries on being Apollo but with Athena window dressing, the tension caused may waste time and lead to some health professionals disengaging from the management task.

So, in summary, Athena is all about hand picking teams to do the job, but within an overall direction, and then letting them get on with the task. Flexible and responsive are the words that come to mind, but as with everything in life, there is a price to be paid.

SELF-REFLECTION 3

Is this what your part of the organisation feels like, or would like to be? Perhaps you work in one of the other cultures but regularly find yourself having to get alongside colleagues who work in an Athena way. Take a moment to note down what happens in these Athena cultures, how it affects your work and, perhaps, why your previous attempts to influence Athena people may not have worked.

DIONYSUS

In Greek mythology Dionysus has several manifestations, but the one we are interested in was his desire to sit outside the norms of his contemporaries, to do his own thing and play by his own rules. Handy refers to him as the first existentialist, whereas others might less charitably call him selfish or self-indulgent. Harrison's original work casts the Dionysus culture as that of the individual, whereby each person has few obligations to others, apart from respecting freedom and autonomy. This emphasis on the individual seems at odds with the notion of a collective culture, and the image chosen by Handy to represent this culture is equally ambiguous.

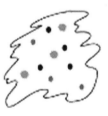

This symbol attempts to show that there is a cohesion and mutual bond within the culture but only at the professional respect level. Its random shape, together with the separation of its elements (the members), remind us that the Dionysus is, at best, a loose collection of individuals.

So how does this culture work, and what clues might tell you that Dionysus is what you have to deal with?

Absolute, unyielding, autonomy

The first and most obvious clue is that the culture is almost always made up of completely autonomous, highly qualified professionals who are used to having their own way. That absolute autonomy may come from their professional code of ethics or from the expectations of their clients. Either way, the average Dionysian is totally self-managed and expects fellow members of the culture to respect that. One might say that there are two rules, both of them unspoken and unwritten, that guide virtually every action taken by members of the Dionysus club.

➤ Rule 1. You can't tell me what to do.
➤ Rule 2. I can't tell you what to do.

Once those two rules are established, Dionysians will happily get on with each other, be curious about each other's practice and, on occasion, pour scorn on each other's ideas, completely safe in the knowledge that none of those behaviours has any real consequence, nor do they set any sort of precedent.

In case you were wondering, Dionysus neatly fits the culture of the body of senior medical staff, and many of our medical clients will quickly and wholeheartedly agree when we explain the model to them!

No structure

In a Dionysus culture, there is no real form or structure to the organisation, and this is normally deliberate. The concept of structure would involve hierarchies, and hierarchies imply seniority and subordination. For Dionysians to adopt either of those roles would immediately compromise one or both of the rules set out earlier. In this culture it is more important to have a little bit of confusion and miscommunication than it is to have a structure that limits professional freedom. This lack of organisational shape means that when members leave or join, the culture just re-forms around them. The icon we use to explain Dionysus is an attempt to represent this fluidity.

Other clues that you are in, or dealing with, a Dionysus culture include:

➤ a general mistrust and avoidance of management processes
➤ a tendency to refer to any necessary management activities as 'administration', thereby lowering its perceived importance
➤ willingness to be extremely robust in criticising and challenging other members of the culture
➤ a refusal by any member to be used as a representative or spokesperson for colleagues (as this again would compromise the two rules)
➤ a tendency to initially find fault with new ideas and approaches, even if members eventually warm to those ideas and adopt them. This is often just a way of reminding others of their complete autonomy – some describe this as 'marking the territory'
➤ a rapid and surprisingly robust solidarity when facing threat from outside. Many influencers have come to grief by thinking that Dionysus' lack of

corporate behaviour makes them easy to pick off one by one. If any Dionysian member feels that what is happening to one may be rolled out to the others, the resultant strength in numbers will almost always lead to victory.

Readers will probably have their own examples of Dionysian triumphs but here are two from our memory.

A health authority was seeking to rationalise a particular clinical service on one site as opposed to the previous two sites, and had entered into service contracts with the appropriate provider organisations. The assumption was that the medical and nursing staff would move sites, but for various reasons, this was rejected by the medics involved. A potential consequence of that impasse was that the employment contracts of those involved would then be terminated as the hospital they worked at would no longer have a service for them to deliver. As word spread among the Dionysus community, instant meetings amongst senior medical staff, most of whom had no interest in the clinical specialty of their affected colleagues, produced a vote of no confidence in the entire Board. High-level intervention failed to resolve the issue and within days several Board and executive members had resigned. Dionysus then returned to its normal loose coalition state with no loss of membership.

One of us carried out a piece of facilitation work with a project team set up to improve theatre throughput at a major hospital. On that group was a consultant anaesthetist who was both interested in the work of the group and keen to help where possible. As the research phase was completed it became clear to all that starting lists on time would be a 'quick win'. Having identified that other commitments amongst the anaesthetists were delaying the start, everyone agreed that if those could be rearranged everyone could be ready to start much earlier. The anaesthetist present quickly agreed to change his schedule accordingly and the meeting sensed a resolution. However, when asked to inform his colleagues of the new arrangement, he declined as he was not acting as any sort of spokesperson or mandated representative. Optimism turned to frustration and then outright incredulity when the doctor concerned pointed out that if his colleagues all wanted to carry on with that other work and continue arriving in theatre later, he would defend absolutely their right to do so.

What the group had failed to spot was that, whilst they all represented cultures where hierarchies and delegated decision-making powers were in place, no one could adopt such a role for Dionysus. The meeting broke up in acrimony, with other team members accusing the medical staff of deliberately sabotaging a perfectly good idea. The resultant damage to goodwill took time to reverse, all because of clash of cultures and the belief, mentioned earlier, that people are either like us, or they jolly well should be.

Curiosity

The final characteristic of Dionysus, and one of great use to the would-be influencer, is that Dionysians are endlessly curious. Their professional interest drives them to look at new things and turn them over in their mind, even if, as mentioned earlier, their initial reaction is to pour cold water over the proposal. There is an unspoken competitiveness between Dionysus members that has them looking over the wall at what their colleagues are up to and wanting to do better. Sometimes that leaks out into the less than polite critiquing of each other's abilities. We have heard Dionysians utter phrases like 'That's rubbish, it will never work, you're insane, which idiot came up with that, you won't catch me following suit', etc. Often, a little while later, when the showboating has finished, you might see a more reflective conversation along the lines of 'I still think it's crazy but tell me more about that idea of yours'. It seems that, as long as the 'two rules' have been re-emphasised, the conversation settles down into a chat between two people who respect each other and share the same value set. Casual, uninformed onlookers may simply see two people with short fuses, open contempt, and little chance of working together.

Although we have spotlighted the medical body as a good example of Dionysus, this culture can also be found in other high-status, high-autonomy professions such as architecture, accountancy and the law. It seems that where professional competence has to be high, and there is a public demand that those professionals are free to do what is best for the client/patient in front of them, it is likely that a Dionysus culture will be in place.

SELF-REFLECTION 4

Just before we outline how best to go about influencing these various cultures, take a final moment to assess whether the people and teams you are trying to get alongside represent Dionysus. Are they on your radar? Do you have to work with them on a regular basis and get them on board with new ideas? If so, how did it go last time, and what have you picked up from our descriptions that might help explain the result you achieved?

APPROACHES THAT WORK (IN THE RIGHT PLACE AND TIME!)

Once you are clear which culture or cultures you are working with, then you can build up specific and targeted influencing strategies for each occasion. As you read on, it is important for us to point out that the approaches that might work for one culture will almost certainly fail with any of the others. We have already highlighted that we are often unaware of our own *default* approaches. However, because they *are* our default settings, we simply assume that everyone else will connect with our arguments and our style of delivery, *or that they should do if they know what's best for them!*

The smart influencer realises that he or she is dealing with different people and cultures, and adapts their style accordingly. The unthinking influencer operates on the principle that (a bit like being a Brit on holiday) if they slow down and speak a little louder, the locals will eventually understand them.

Here, then, are the approaches that will work for the smart influencer. The following table summarises the four sets of approaches so that you can immediately see the contrasts. What then follows is greater detail on each one.

WITH A ZEUS CULTURE	WITH AN APOLLO CULTURE
➤ Find out what is on Zeus' agenda	➤ Work carefully with, and honour, the evidence
➤ Offer solutions, not additional complex problems	➤ Show detailed planning and full risk appraisal
➤ Allow Zeus to adopt, and bask in, the idea	➤ Put things down on paper
➤ Keep it simple and direct	➤ Allow and promote consultation and cautious consideration
➤ Focus on success and impact	➤ Take time, and allow for time
➤ Work with the inner circle (they know the timing and the language to use)	➤ Use the proper channels
➤ Don't argue until you are seen as credible	➤ Cover all options and demonstrate transparency in the decision-making process
➤ Find the prodigal sons within the organisation, those who are currently in favour, and work with them	➤ Respect hierarchy and committee processes

WITH AN ATHENA CULTURE	WITH A DIONYSUS CULTURE
➤ Honour the personal skills of those involved	➤ Avoid corporate initiatives and rolled-out programmes
➤ Demonstrate trust in those individuals	➤ Establish personal credibility with one or two members of the culture
➤ Pick the team for the job	➤ Work with them and allow the results to speak for themselves
➤ Delegate ruthlessly	
➤ Tap into a professional desire to do the best that can be done	➤ Avoid elaborate management mechanisms
➤ Be clear about endpoints, then step back	➤ Acknowledge professional freedom to slow down, opt out, change direction, re-engage, etc.
➤ Encourage free communication, unconstrained by 'usual channels'	➤ Offer help rather than seeking compliance
➤ Reward achievements quickly, vocally and innovatively	➤ Build up a subject expertise that others are free to use if desired
	➤ Accept initial suspicion as the norm

Influencing the Zeus culture

The key words here are *simplicity, impact, personal and 'inner circle'*. You now know that the Zeus culture revolves around the personal, and often unpredictable, wishes of the central Zeus character. Quite simply, unless the proposal you want to make is to the point, good for Zeus (personally as well as workwise) and contains all the key words that get their attention quickly, you could be doing more harm than good.

One of us worked, briefly, for a Zeus character who delighted in unsettling callers to his office by looking sternly over his half-rim glasses and barking 'You have 5 minutes – what do you want?'. Suffice to say people only went in there unprepared once!

Do not be fooled into thinking that Zeus characters are dense or have limited intellectual powers. They are often supremely intelligent and may be simply choosing to spend a short time on your issue because they have so many other issues to grapple with. Therefore do not interpret *simple* as meaning 'dumbed down'. Even if your 'pitch' is simple and to the point, you need to have all the background facts at your disposal, in case Zeus gets absorbed and wants to dig deeper.

One way to look at this is to imagine what you would have in front of you and what is tucked behind your back, just in case.

For Zeus, the impact comes first, like so!

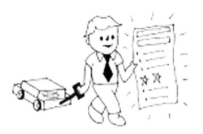

Never go near the Zeus character until you have done your research. Find out what is currently keeping them awake at night, or what they are constantly exhorting their staff to do, then customise your proposal to be something that will help move one of those issues forward. Otherwise you will simply be seen as adding to the agenda rather than taking something off it!

Finding out the topics is one thing, but you also need to find out when would be a good time, and what language to avoid or use. For this, the inner circle comes into play. Indeed, there may be times when you need to set your sights lower than Zeus and settle for getting alongside one of the current inner circle instead. They will know what works and what doesn't, can answer questions on timing and style, and may even take up your idea and speak directly to Zeus on your behalf.

Some years ago, one of us needed the CEO of a health trust to endorse a programme we were running and to agree to speak to the participants. Clearly, we needed to demonstrate value for money, the likelihood of impact, and flatter him enough for him to open up a slot in his diary. At the time we were virtually unknown to the man, let alone on his current radar, and any formal meeting to put forward the proposal would have been difficult to arrange and held under a great deal of pressure. Fortunately we had access to another of the trust's executive team, someone who we had already worked with, and we met her to rehearse our thinking. The result was that she offered to 'have a word', citing a forthcoming long car journey she was to share with the CEO, and she agreed to connect the programme with Zeus' current concern about the way managers were perceived by senior clinicians in the trust. Two weeks later we got a call saying 'Go ahead, he's on board and in fact he will be coming to several sessions just to show his commitment'. In fact, the first time we actually met the CEO was at one of those sessions but, by then, we had got what we wanted! However, we had to share the limelight.

As this story shows, one of the prices you may have to pay for getting Zeus on your side is that the idea may be adopted by Zeus and sometimes blatantly publicised as theirs. The first time this happened to one of us, it provoked mixed emotions. Obviously, we were pleased to be getting the idea or proposal off the ground but, after all, it was our idea and the thought of Zeus standing on various platforms basking in the feedback was quite hard to take. This hijacking of others' ideas is often innocent and accidental and seems to just be part of this lack of separation between Zeus the person and their organisation. When they say 'We are ...', they may mean 'I am ...', and when they say 'I am ...' they could be meaning 'We are ...'.

This means that the smart influencer will need on occasion to suppress their own ego on the basis that getting the right decision is more important than being in the spotlight.

If you can get direct to Zeus, then go ahead, but look for the informal as well as the formal opportunities. It sounds a bit of a caricature to talk about deals being done on the golf course, but a receptive Zeus is often to be found in 'non-office' settings, and the smart influencer will take advantage of those situations. Don't worry so much about whether you will be seen as underhand or resorting to lobbying. As long as you have done your research, get to the point and demonstrate personal credibility, you will get a hearing. You may even be surprised to get a decision straight away, so anticipate the question 'If I say yes, how soon can this be up and running?'.

Influencing the Apollo culture

Glance again at the list of Zeus influencing approaches and then ignore them. If you try any of them when talking to the Apollo culture, you are doomed to failure *and* a deteriorating reputation. Getting straight to the point, particularly if you are painting the big picture and the future state, makes Apollo uneasy due to the lack of evidence and your failure to have first established the case for change.

In contrast to the high-impact nature of your pitch to Zeus (backed up by the evidence if needed), Apollo wants first to be reassured that this is a serious matter and has been subject to serious consideration. In short, the data come first, as the picture below clearly shows.

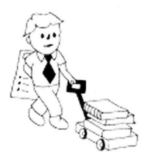

As you can see from the earlier table, Apollo likes evidence, analysis and soundness of planning. The overall impression is one of thoughtfulness, and typical Apollonians respond well to those who demonstrate a similar respect for cautious consideration. Put quite simply, Apollo will not be rushed, however frustrated you might become as a result. In their world, rushed decisions are bad decisions, bad decisions carry risk, and Apollo is risk averse.

It is important to take on board that the *form* of your influencing has to be as thorough as the case itself.

> One of us undertook a piece of work for a government department some years ago, the product of which was a report with recommendations for significant changes in health strategy in that area. The draft version was returned with the request that the report be made longer! Apparently, given the significance of the recommendations and the seniority of those who were to read the document, the report needed to have more gravitas and authority – it needed, quite literally, more 'weight'. A desire for brevity would have been welcomed in our own culture but in Apollo, brevity could be interpreted as insufficient rigour.

Readers outside this culture may look at this story with incredulity and ill-disguised contempt, but it will do you no good. If you want Apollo to come on board with your ideas and proposals, you will need to do things their way. After all, that is what you would like from those trying to influence you.

We have already mentioned Apollo and risk. For this reason, any proposal that does not contain a detailed risk analysis or option appraisal is likely to be politely but firmly ignored. Not only does option appraisal tick the box of demonstrating rigour, it also lays out the pros and cons of all the various ideas, not just the one you are proposing. The better you are at playing down personal ownership of your favoured plan, ironically the more Apollo will trust your analysis. Influencers are sometimes guilty of blatantly loading their favoured option in the way they pick and then score the various appraisal criteria and this simply causes Apollo to mistrust the whole process. Critical point: once objectivity is lost, Apollo gets worried. In contrast, once subjectivity and personal passion are lost, Zeus loses interest. Hence our emphasis on picking the right approach for the culture and not trying to use the same approach with different cultures.

Also, never forget to cover the implications of doing nothing. For Apollo, the do nothing option is always on the table unless you can show that such a choice is unwise. Zeus, on the other hand, is programmed to do stuff so don't waste time on such analysis.

Another sharp contrast between Zeus and Apollo is that, whilst the former will not be fazed by informal and innovative ways of making contact, protocol and procedure are vital to the latter and those who undermine due process are viewed with suspicion. Take time to find out who has the power to say yes, and then approach them formally. If there is a committee with a remit that covers your idea, approach the chair or secretary and take their advice on how and when to put forward your proposal.

If there is an annual planning cycle (bids received in November, evaluated in December, and budgets set in February, etc.), honour this and time your submission accordingly. Don't send in something in May and demand that it is considered there and then.

Another important piece of protocol to bear in mind. The person you speak to to get information and research is probably not the decision maker so don't place them in the awkward position of making decisions above their level of authority. In Zeus cultures, as long as the person you are speaking to knows exactly what Zeus will/won't support, you may get a quick decision, but the structures of Apollo militate against this speed of decision making.

Just as Zeus will have pet projects and current 'flavours of the month', Apollo will have policies, strategies and plans. The main difference is that the latter are likely to be more stable and long-lasting. One way to get Apollo really interested in your proposal is to link it to one or more of the strategies or policy initiatives that are already on the books. If your proposal document shows how your plan fits into the current direction of travel, this will raise its profile.

This is an example form of words that make those connections.

> The XYZ Health Board has already made a public commitment to give patients a greater say in how local services are delivered and the recently launched strategy 'Using both ears to hear our patients' sets out some ambitious targets for improving patient involvement. Our proposal to pilot web-based patient forums would make a significant contribution to target 5 of the strategy and we would like to work with your patient involvement department to ensure that our work is fully integrated with existing activities.

Clearly this is just an example, but it has been deliberately worded to pick up some important themes – connection, targets, contribution, working together, acknowledging others in the field, etc. Your research will tell you what the key strategies and drivers are for your target culture and then you can make the connections for yourself.

If there are no connections to be made, then don't try, as this would look contrived, but you will need to work harder to get Apollo to see the need to consider your proposal separately. The best way of doing this is to show, legally and ethically, that the risks of not looking at your proposal are greater than the risks of doing so. This way, you are still working with the grain of that culture (risk assessment) but also addressing their tendency to see the do nothing option as always available.

Influencing the Athena culture

The summary table above reminds us that Athenians are practical in nature and 'team friendly' in organisational terms. They like a challenge, the freedom to innovate and the permission to self-manage. They welcome co-workers who bring complementary skills to the party, regardless of grade and history, and their allegiances tend to be to the project or projects they are working on rather than to a figurehead or an organisational identity. For those used to working in Zeus or Apollo cultures, it can be a real challenge to adopt behaviours that help get alongside Athena but, as with the others, any failure to adapt will result in a failure to persuade.

These hints suggest that the critical thing with Athena is to *involve them early* in shaping both the issues that you need them to work on and the way in which they will be able to work. The best way to do this is for you to approach and handpick the person you would like to lead or co-ordinate the work, tell them they have been approached because of their skills and achievements, set them a real and exciting challenge and allow them to handpick the people they would like to work with.

By all means let them know what the overall direction and desired outcomes will be, clearly state any negotiables and constraints, but then get out of the way and let these people get on with it. From that moment on your role is to support, open doors outside the organisation if necessary, speak warmly about the team in high places, and secure resources as and when needed. What you must not do with Athena is say and do all those things at the start and then begin to micromanage, particularly if things are getting sensitive or tricky. Zeus culture members may find this difficult as they suspect that Zeus will not want to let go and will demand to know that things are going the way they want, and Apollonians are too used to setting up groups with clear remits, terms of reference, etc., with elaborate reporting arrangements back to the parent committee. Once Athena feels untrusted or hemmed in by over-engineered reporting mechanisms, their commitment and enthusiasm for the task wane and they will seek their professional satisfaction from their other projects.

Having got Athena interested and keen to help, an additional challenge for the influencer is to allow creativity in both how the work is tackled and how the team works and communicates. It is not unusual for Athena organisations to have a less than rigid approach to working hours, use of professional titles, multi-tasking and line management relationships. For example, we know of one Athena culture where the project team approach is so flexible that manager A can be a member of one work team, leader of another, and a technical contributor to a third team whose leader is one of their own subordinate staff. Try maintaining any sort of traditional hierarchical reporting arrangements there and the team members will simply look baffled. If you are someone who can be clear about ends and extremely flexible about means (by which we mean innovative, not unethical), you will find it easier to get on the same wavelength as Athena.

Influencing the Dionysus culture

You will recall that Dionysus is the culture of the self-managed individual, where professional autonomy is not only sought – it is demanded. Anything that might potentially conflict with or compromise that freedom is ruthlessly rejected, even if (in the eyes of others) the idea being offered is sound and the decision to say no has overtones of sabotage. This is not the right place to debate the rights and wrongs of any culture's operating principles – readers just have to accept for now that this is how Dionysus works.

They key to successful influencing with this culture is to stop seeing it as having any collective identity. See it instead as a group of individuals who, *as individuals*, might be interested in working with you on your idea or proposal. Then approach one of them (having done some research as to who might be open to a discussion) and simply set out some ideas. However, and this is absolutely vital, do not see this conversation as the start of a roll-out campaign to the other Dionysians. Treat it as simply the start of a possible collaboration with that individual alone.

If you give the impression that you are simply starting with the 'line of least resistance' and that the rest of the culture will be next, one of two things will almost certainly happen.

➤ The first is that the person you are speaking to will withdraw for fear of being seen by colleagues as some sort of management stooge.

➤ The second is that the rest of the culture will either distance itself from the person you are speaking to or will actively seek to undermine the project by other means.

It is critical that you protect the person you are speaking to by making it clear to them, and anyone else who asks, that this work is a collaborative project between two people with no hidden agenda and no planned roll-out. A typical form of words might be:

> Dr X and I are working on a new way of treating condition Y, and the results are encouraging so far. If you want any more information on what we are doing and why, come and see us but otherwise this is a discrete and small-scale project.

Of course, this has to be true, so don't try this if you do have a hidden agenda. When you are found out, and you will be, the cherished reputation we talk about so much in this book will be in tatters.

Once you have reassured all concerned that this is what it looks like – a genuine attempt to work with one professional and solve a shared problem – your job is done. What will happen over time is that Dionysus' innate curiosity will lead to an increase in conversations between members. In other words, the work you are doing will spread virally, and a few more members will make contact, either with you or with their colleague. At this point, do not be surprised if this contact is highly sceptical or negative. We have experienced contact from Dionysians along the lines of: 'I hear you are working with X. Sounds flaky to me and I'm sure these results won't transfer to my area of practice. (Later ...) However, I wouldn't mind getting some more information about it'.

What is going on here is a clear restatement of the two rules governing Dionysus cultures, coupled with a desire not to be left behind if anything interesting and innovative is going on. However, the most significant element is that the person is making contact on their own terms. If you had tried to make contact with those other people, your motives would have been questioned and a master plan suspected.

Your role should be to respond with dignity and a genuine desire to help, and make sure that any work you then do with that person is subject to the same terms as applied to the first person – this is a private arrangement between two people and the work does not affect anyone else without their consent.

As you read this, you can be forgiven for thinking 'I haven't got the time to wait that long – I am under pressure from above to get this thing rolled out now'. Our advice is somewhat blunt. We appreciate your dilemma but, from our experience, you will spend much longer coping with the resistance and stalled progress caused by their rejection of a corporate approach than you will sowing seeds and letting the culture do things in its own time. The corporate approach simply does not work, unless you have serious control of the reward or sanction system, and your attempts will damage your reputation for next time. The recommended approach takes time but leads to sustainable change. You decide which method you want to be associated with.

SUMMARY

This is a significant chapter with a considerable amount of research and analysis on the various cultures. We conclude with some key messages and some caveats.

The caveats

Any model of organisational thinking can be useful in that it simplifies and codifies an otherwise complex subject. Models can give us a common language that helps make sense of that complexity. However, almost all models are a gross oversimplification and risk readers trying to fit their own experiences into whichever model the writer might offer. Whatever you think about the usefulness and accessibility of Harrison's original typology of cultures and Handy's development of the model, there are many more cultures around than just these four. Furthermore, not every Zeus culture will fit the pen portrait we offer in this chapter. The same goes for the other three 'gods'.

However, these models do challenge us to think differently. They helpfully remind us that not every team or department is like us and that the things that would make perfect sense to us might mean little or nothing to others. Not because they are less intelligent or less committed, but simply because they work in different ways. If this fundamental point has sunk in then this chapter will have achieved its primary purpose.

The main messages

This chapter is not an invitation to engage in academic 'god spotting'. The labels are far less important than the need to simply step back before you go into influencing mode and think through these questions.

➤ Who am I wanting to get on board?
➤ Where do they work and what might be the legitimate constraints placed by that organisation on how they operate?
➤ If I don't know the answers, what can I do to find out?
➤ Armed with this information and insight, what is the best way I can present my ideas?
➤ Am I the best person to do this or are there others in the team who would simply click with the target audience much more quickly than I could?

As with Chapter 2 on personality, it is important to remember that you will be more successful in influencing others if you go with the grain of how they operate. If you combine new ideas with challenges to their current way of operating, you risk them finding easy reasons to say no. You also risk offending, albeit innocently, their important and cherished rituals. Hardly a good foundation for making your case!

Our view is simple and clear. Differences are good and necessary. Diversity leads to creativity. Yes, it increases the chances of misunderstanding but we think this is a price worth paying. Uniformity and conformity may make management easier at a superficial level, but organisations will only grow and develop if people (and the teams they work in) are allowed to be themselves. Diagnosing and then honouring different organisational cultures is just one way of releasing the potential of those people.

Now you have learned more about all four cultures, and their associated influencing approaches, here is a final opportunity for reflection followed by action.

SELF-REFLECTION 5

Identify one of the work areas or organisations around you, where:

➤ your job success is partly dependent on influencing those who work there, and

➤ so far you have met with mixed success.

Record some tentative conclusions about the prevailing culture or cultures at work in that area (test these out in conversation with others if necessary).

Identify a new set of approaches, based on the advice in this chapter, that would improve your chances next time.

Repeat this reflective process immediately after that 'next time'.

REFERENCES

1 Harrison R. Understanding your organisation's character. *Harvard Bus Rev.* 1972; 5(3): 119–28.
2 Handy C. *Gods of Management.* London: Business Books; 1991.
3 Machiavelli N. *The Prince.* London: Penguin; 1961.

CHAPTER 4

Influencing organisational change

When people talk of the need for change, they are usually thinking that it is someone else who needs to change.

(Richard Axelrod[1])

There's no limit to what a man can achieve, if he doesn't care who gets the credit.

(Laing Burns Jr)

Change in most organisations is treated as a technical exercise. Problems are identified and analysed, statistics studied, options considered and a solution is chosen by a small group of top managers. This solution, usually involving new organisational structures or systems, is then announced. Staff are expected to enthusiastically embrace a solution they have had no part in designing. If they express other views they are seen as difficult. To encourage compliance, managers use a variety of carrot and stick (but mainly stick!) approaches. The sudden blitz of consultations, presentations and newsletters that accompany organisational upheaval will be familiar to almost anyone who has worked in healthcare. But in most cases, the hoped-for transformation in quality or performance never quite happens and the fallout from the changes rumbles on for months or years. Then, two or three years later another initiative is launched to address the lack of progress and the pattern is repeated.

This chapter argues that it is our failure to see change as a human as well as a technical process that causes the depressing cycle described above. We'll look at some evidence about the effectiveness of the usual approach to change and then examine its origins in what is sometimes called Scientific Management. We'll then suggest that we need to fundamentally rethink organisational change and recognise that it is largely concerned with people. Finally, we'll offer some guidelines for facilitating change whether you have organisational authority or just the opportunity to influence.

CHANGE: THE EVIDENCE

Consider this: most organisational change programmes go partly or completely wrong, and the main cause of this is how we deal with the people involved. Estimates of exactly how often change fails vary but tend to cluster around 60–70%.[2,3] One recent survey of over 1500 managers from Europe, Asia and the Americas[4] found that:

➤ just 41% of projects succeeded in meeting their objectives, on time and in budget
➤ 59% missed one objective or failed entirely
➤ the best companies had an 80% success rate, the worst 8%
➤ the biggest challenges were not resources or technology, but the culture, mindsets and attitudes of the people involved.

Even with this worrying failure rate our appetite for major change programmes, particularly reorganisations, remains undiminished. A 2003 survey of UK private and public sector organisations found that many embarked on major changes every two to three years despite the fact that 'around half of reorganisations fail to meet their objectives, take longer to implement than planned and cost more than budgeted. In some cases reorganisations have no impact at all or even make matters worse'.[5] The survey also confirmed that how people were treated was a critical factor in determining success or failure.

The evidence is clear. The idea that organisations successfully change shape or direction on the basis of orders from above is largely fictional. The uncomfortable truth is that we are not good at achieving the change we want in organisations. The normal top-down, command and control approach is, it turns out, very ineffective. Indeed, 'evidence that top management has the power to drive change efforts is thin, at best'.[6] It is also clear that the main reason for this is the way we deal with people. People – involving them, talking with them, listening to them – are at the heart of change. Our failure to grasp this lies behind most of the problems we encounter.

EVERYTHING WE KNOW IS WRONG

It may seem odd that managers persist in managing change in a way that usually fails. To understand why, we need to see that this is largely the result of widespread beliefs about people and organisations which have been accepted as true, but which are at best questionable. Many of these beliefs have their roots in the work of F.W. Taylor, an engineer born in 1856 in Germantown, Pennsylvania. He developed his ideas while working as chief engineer in a steelworks and then manager of a paper mill. In these large industrial settings, he saw the problem as being how to raise everyone's performance to the level of the most productive worker. Taylor's approach was to try to control work in the way that an engineer might control a machine.[7] Every task was broken down into its constituent parts and analysed to arrive at the best, most efficient way of doing the job. Scientific Management, as this approach became known, very deliberately sought to remove from the individual worker the capacity to make judgements about what to do and how to do it. Instead of leaving things to the craft and know-how of the employee, management would use scientific principles to determine the best way for work to be done.

Seeing organisations as machines resulted in managers seeing themselves as engineers whose task was to operate, repair or upgrade the machine. In this paradigm, the employee was a component who should perform within specified tolerances (job descriptions and objectives). If change was required, faulty components (people) could be mended (retrained) or replaced (sacked). Initiative and innovation were not required as these were the prerogative of the manager, assisted by consultants and work-study specialists, who would measure and analyse work processes in order to remove waste and increase efficiency.

It is easy to see the full flowering of Scientific Management in public sector bureaucracies where every procedure is standardised and staff are carefully graded and fitted into predetermined slots in rigid hierarchies. Indeed, many healthcare organisations are run in this way. But the influence of Scientific Management is no less present in private sector companies which see themselves as much more go-ahead but share this view of the organisation as a machine which must be controlled. One clue about the prevailing management philosophy in such organisations is the way the language is often drawn from physics and engineering. Employees who think independently are 'resistors', teams are 're-engineered' and change is 'kick-started' or 'driven' through. What underpins organisations who, knowingly or unknowingly, embrace Scientific Management are beliefs such as:

➤ change comes from the top
➤ money is the supreme motivator
➤ we need strong leaders to force change through
➤ people will resist change
➤ efficiency comes from control.

Even in Taylor's day, Scientific Management was criticised for deskilling the workforce. Its principles assumed a largely uneducated workforce, motivated only by money. But today its flaws are even more apparent. The employee is dehumanised and discouraged from thinking beyond her job description and a cautious passivity is induced by management's attempt to standardise and proceduralise every aspect of her work. The belief that change must be pushed through and that it will be resisted by the workforce becomes a self-fulfilling prophecy as attempts by managers to force change upon employees create an understandably negative reaction.

This approach to change, where a small group of senior managers initiate, direct and control the changes with little attempt to involve staff, has been found to fail more often than not.[8] Nevertheless, it continues to be the default style in many organisations. It is born out of the pervasive Scientific Management view of organisations as machines and people as components.

PEOPLE, AUTHORITY AND CHANGE

As this book was being written, what has been called the 'Arab Spring' dominated the news. Large numbers of people in countries such as Egypt, Libya and Syria were demanding more of a say in how their communities were shaped and governed. The people participating in these movements often did so at the cost of their lives or freedom. Despite the overwhelming military force at their disposal, those in charge found it difficult, and in several cases impossible, to impose their will.

Such events are an extreme but potent reminder of the human desire to have a say in decisions that affect us and of the surprising impotence of sheer force to suppress this desire. They also underline the fact that having formal authority, political or organisational, does not guarantee success in times of change.

Although many managers would not recognise the name of F.W. Taylor or the term 'Scientific Management', Taylor's principles have become so deeply ingrained in the theory and practice of management that they are no more likely to be questioned than the roundness of the earth or the existence of gravity. This mechanistic view of organisations is an example of a mental model (see Chapter 1) which inhibits learning. Taylor's views, which were in their day a contentious break with the past, calling for a 'complete mental revolution',[9] are now the orthodoxy. Unfortunately they lead to managers attempting to create change in ways that are prone to failure. Another mental revolution is required.

THE NEED FOR A RETHINK

Henry Ford, a disciple of Taylor, once lamented: 'Why is it every time I ask for a pair of hands, they come with a brain attached?'. People's capacity to think independently and their desire for self-determination are a problem for top-down managers that has to be overcome by carrots such as money or promotion or sticks such as the disciplinary procedure or the threat of redundancy. But what if this capacity for independent thought were a potential advantage? What if the intelligence and energy of the workforce that sometimes hinder conventional change approaches could be in themselves a source of innovation and improvement?

For many years the big question in change management has been 'how can we overcome staff resistance?'. To this end managers have dazzled staff with Power-Point, herded them into stage-managed consultations and browbeaten them with surveys and consultants' reports. But it is fundamentally the wrong question. We should be asking, 'how can we make staff part of the change process?'. This is especially the case in healthcare organisations where so many of our staff see their work as more than just a job. Rather than seeing staff as a complicating factor, we need to see them as our greatest asset in improving the way healthcare is provided.

THE HUMANITY OF ORGANISATIONS

It sounds obvious when we say that organisations are made up of people, not parts. But this recognition brings about a profound shift in our approach to change. Scientific Management, with its machine thinking, leads many managers to treat change as if it were a mechanical problem. Thinking of the organisation as an impersonal, inanimate object leads to managers acting as if the laws of classical physics apply and mass, force and velocity are critical. In this way of thinking, changing a large organisation will require a large change project or smaller swifter projects.[3] Overcoming resistance will require even greater force. But this approach is revealed as inappropriate and often counterproductive when we remember that an organisation is primarily people, all of whom have the capacity to make choices, to be inspired or bored, to co-operate or to sabotage depending on how they are treated.

THE HUMAN ORGANISATION

For the first time since the dawning of the industrial age, the only way to build a company that's fit for the future is to build one that's fit for human beings as well. This is your opportunity – to build a 21st century management model that truly elicits, honours and cherishes human initiative, creativity, and passion ... Do this and you will have built an organisation that is fully human and fully prepared for the extraordinary opportunities that lie ahead.[10]

Gary Hamel, Visiting Professor of Strategic and International Management, London Business School.

What do we know about people at work? Let's start with someone you know well: yourself. Think for a moment about your experiences as an employee. Focus on the times when you have been at your best, the times when you have willingly put your heart and soul into your work and wanted to find new ways to get better results. Now think about how you felt about your work and your colleagues at those times.

It's likely that you felt trusted[11] and supported by your boss and that he or she had high expectations of you. You probably felt that you had a valuable[12] part to play in your team and that, because of this, you did not want to let anyone down. Also, you were likely to have had a sense of purpose or meaning in your work, a vision[13] you were pursuing or a feeling that your work was worthwhile and interesting. This is the mix of factors that results in enthusiastic, committed staff who, far from resisting change, are open to innovation.

Feeling trusted and valued and having a sense of purpose and vision are all things which are largely determined by relationships in the workplace and how managers treat their staff. Wise managers build a climate of trust where staff feel valued. They do so by action and example. We have heard managers defend themselves by saying that when their staff act as though they can be trusted, then they will trust them. But such an attitude locks both parties into a cycle of suspicion and poor performance. Instead, the manager has to be the first to show trust. Our reluctance to do so comes in part from the belief that, without controls, people will do the minimum or act irresponsibly. Clocking-in systems, security checks and countersigning testify to a persistent belief that 'they' would act corruptly unless prevented from doing so. We ourselves would be insulted if someone accused us of this. Our point is that most people are like you; managed well, they are capable of doing great work and enthusiastically adopting improvements. It is poor management that is mainly to blame for demotivated, inflexible staff.

Acknowledging the power of being trusted, valued and having a sense of purpose is a far cry from the traditional view of staff as being primarily motivated by greed or fear. Yet its truth is borne out both by research and by reflecting on our own experience in work. Staff managed in this way do not need to be coerced into change. People at work have the potential to do the same things they do outside work, organising themselves and making difficult choices without close supervision. It is a sobering thought that people who successfully raise children, run domestic budgets, manage Boy Scout troops and take evening classes to expand their learning are treated, when they come to work, as if they were unable to think through anything for themselves. Their tasks are proceduralised, their time is controlled and their work is closely monitored. Is it any wonder that, in such circumstances, morale is low and flexibility is a problem? The answer is not more controls and coercion but a revolution in management thinking, a recognition that the organisation is not a machine but a complex social system, a community with a purpose, a network of people. This means that there are significant differences between change in organisations and mechanical change. Perhaps the three most important are:

➤ change is a process, not an event
➤ change is holistic – changes in one part affect the other parts
➤ unlike machines, people can initiate change themselves.

Change is a process

It is because of the humanity of the organisation that the process of change takes on a much greater prominence. There are two reasons for this.

➤ **People take time to change**. For a machine, change is an event. It goes from one gear to the next or from on to off in a moment. People, on the other hand, take time to adjust to change, even when the change is one that they welcome.

➤ **The process of change may be more important than the content**. Managers tend to fixate on the solution: getting the right organisational structure or the right office layout. The process of change is seen as a secondary issue. But even the best solution will falter or fail if the change process leaves staff feeling that they have no voice and no choice. It's worth remembering that with goodwill people can make almost any system work, whereas without it even the best designed system will grind to a halt.

William Bridges[14] makes the point that when people go through major change, they move through a process rather than simply switching from one state to another. He distinguishes between changes and transitions, arguing that *changes* are situational: moving to a new office or taking on new duties, whereas *transitions* are psychological: a process that people experience as they gradually internalise and adapt to a new situation. For example, think of the last time you moved job. Although there was a particular date when one contract ended and a new one began, psychologically and emotionally the process took much longer. In your last days in the old job you may have experienced a mix of anticipation of the new and sadness at the relationships you would be leaving behind. Arriving at your new workplace, your excitement at promotion may have been mingled with nervousness about whether your new colleagues would accept or respect you. Building relationships and learning the unwritten rules that exist in any workplace take time, and during this period you may have looked back with fondness on the team and role you knew so well. The result of all this is that it can take weeks or months to settle down in a new job and feel that you are fully effective. Unlike machines, where the new part – a new lightbulb perhaps – immediately functions at full capacity in its new location, humans experience a gradual transition. We can act in ways which either smooth this transition or prolong it but to ignore it is foolish. Bridges suggests that the process of transition has three overlapping phases.

Phase one: ending, losing, letting go

For something new to start, something old has to end. Even when we initiate something new ourselves, or when the logical case for change is overwhelming, we may still experience a sense of loss or sadness at the breaking up of a team we enjoyed working in or the leaving of a workplace where we spent many years. One of Bridges' suggestions for helping people let go of the old is to treat the past with respect.

Some years ago, a city hospital was scheduled for closure. Patient services were to be moved from the old Victorian building to a new location much better suited to the technological demands of modern medicine. The old hospital was badly located, too small and its support systems were collapsing. The new hospital had far better transport links and brand new wards and theatres. In the process of moving from one to the other, the sole management message was how good the new building would be. If the old building was mentioned, it was only to denigrate it. As the move progressed, the old building was neglected and routine upkeep was reduced or stopped. Despite the clear advantages of the new hospital, many staff moved grudgingly and for years after complained about the new hospital. Management were taken by surprise by the amount of resistance to the move and the hostility towards the new building. Instead of a positive move to a better future, it became tinged with resentment and hindered by foot-dragging. And of course, in a purely logical world this made no sense whatsoever. But what had been forgotten were the years that many staff had spent at the old building, training, working and caring for patients. They had met friends and partners and experienced the unique highs and lows of hospital life all in the outdated, but much loved, corridors of the old hospital. By ignoring all this, by running down the past in a misguided attempt to make the future look even more attractive, management made change much harder than it needed to be.

This attachment to the past may apply to buildings, teams or work routines. It can even apply to the names, logos and titles that provide employees with a sense of identity. One of us once talked with managers from an insurance company that, upon being taken over by a USA business, had lost its traditional company emblem, a squirrel. The new bosses were perplexed by the energetic, grass-roots 'save the squirrel' campaign that came, seemingly, from nowhere. Issues like identity, memory and pride cannot be measured and will not appear on a balance sheet but they certainly influence the behaviour of people at work. The wise manager treats the past with respect and accepts the sense of loss that staff may feel even if he or she does not share it. We should not be thrown when staff display anger or sadness when old ways of working are coming to an end. This will be the case even when those same staff accept the logic or inevitability of change. Alongside carefully making the case for change, acknowledging their loss and honouring the past can help them let go and move on. One training organisation we know marked its renaming and restructuring by holding an event to remember its greatest successes. Having celebrated the past, staff were able to confidently move on, bringing with them all that was good about the old organisation. Such techniques accelerate, rather than draw out, the inevitable transition process.

> ### INDIVIDUAL TRANSITIONS
>
> The idea that people go through a transition process in response to major life changes is already widely accepted in relation to individuals. As long ago as 1969, Elisabeth Kübler-Ross[15] set out her 'five stages of grief' model, based on research with dying patients, which has since been applied to other experiences such as being made redundant. While the familiar denial-anger-bargaining-depression-acceptance model has its critics, it highlights an important truth in relation to how we undergo major change. The same understanding also needs to be applied to how groups of people in organisations experience major change.

Phase two: the neutral zone

To illustrate what is meant by the neutral zone, let's return to the experience of starting a new job. In the first days and weeks, although you already have the technical know-how you need, so much is new and unfamiliar. In your last job you had an established place in the pecking order and a set of friends. You knew who really had the power to make things happen and you were comfortably familiar with the hundreds of little rituals that add up to an organisation's culture, such as how meetings are run, how people speak to each other and even dress code. Now, none of this makes sense any more and you have yet to learn the new rules. Misunderstandings and confusion threaten and you have to learn fast. As a result, you may feel more anxious and a little less confident than usual. Welcome to the neutral zone, where the old ways no longer work and the new ways are still unclear. It's a time when people feel disoriented by the disappearance of old certainties and much of their energy is diverted into coping with this. During this phase people may become defensive, and the ongoing uncertainty will inevitably lower their effectiveness. The discomfort produced by ambiguity will result in some people wishing they could return to the comfort of familiar roles and relationships.

One health organisation unintentionally made the neutral zone almost unbearable for its staff by prolonging uncertainty during an organisational restructuring. After the old organisational structures were pronounced unfit for purpose, months went by before the new structures were approved and announced. During this time rumour proliferated and in the absence of trusted briefings from management, staff were ready to believe the worst about their future prospects. As if this were not bad enough, the process of selecting staff for the new jobs was ponderously slow, lasting well over a year. The hidden cost of this in terms of sickness, loss of goodwill and the impact on the families of those concerned was enormous.

The neutral zone is a necessary part of change. It's the place where we leave behind old patterns of working and begin to develop new ways, new networks, new perspectives. For this reason it can be a creative place where old habits and assumptions can make way for fresh ideas. But there is much we can do to help people through this zone rather than letting them wander round in the wilderness without vision or direction. The first thing is to prepare staff for the experience, because most will expect to simply move from the old to the new. Let them know that it is normal for there to be a period of readjustment and that it will take time for the new structure/IT system/team to settle down. We can also help by keeping people well informed. And don't fall into the trap of only communicating with your staff where there is something to announce. Nature abhors a vacuum, and your silence will be quickly filled by rumour and speculation. During a period of change, communicate regularly even if it is to say that there is nothing to say! If possible, use meetings, training and other events to strengthen connections in the work group and help minimise feelings of isolation. Finally, make the most of the creative potential of the neutral zone. If you are building a new team or settling into new accommodation, encourage innovation and promote new, more effective work processes.

MOSES AND THE NEUTRAL ZONE

In his book *Managing Transitions*, William Bridges uses the biblical story of Moses and the exodus to illustrate the dangers of the neutral zone.[14] Having gladly left a life of slavery in Egypt, the Israelites then find that they must cross a wilderness before reaching the Promised Land. The rebellions and grumbling Moses had to cope with and the way the Israelites began to idealise the past will be familiar to any manager who has led people into unfamiliar territory. Moses learned to his cost that while it didn't take long to get the people out of Egypt, it took a long time to get Egypt out of the people. But it was only in the wilderness that Moses was able to establish the new culture and sense of identity that would turn a collection of slaves into a nation.

Phase three: new beginnings

Any new system or new structure will have a particular start date but we should not assume that this is when staff will experience a new beginning. The new beginning is when, having let go of the past and negotiated the neutral zone, people embrace the new processes, values and perspectives that the change was designed to bring about. This is when the new team or new structure begins to achieve its potential and when the new system begins to work smoothly.

Because the new beginning depends on moving through the other two phases, some transitions never make it this far. Superficially, the change has taken place but the hoped-for benefits never quite materialise. Instead of the bright future envisaged in the consultant's report, old habits and old problems hang around like unwelcome guests who won't leave the party. But before announcing another reorganisation or blaming the new software, we would be well advised to reflect for a moment. Bridges' three-phase model helps us understand that the problem in cases like this may not be with the change itself but with the way we helped, or failed to help, people through the transition process.

Many health organisations have attempted to delegate decision making to clinical departments, giving them the freedom to manage staffing and budgets in a way that makes sense for their patients. It is common for these experiments to be abandoned after a few years, usually when the clinicians find that they have a good deal less freedom than they thought. There is much to commend the idea of such delegation, but it requires a transition. Old ideas about central control and the roles of managers and clinicians need to be jettisoned and there needs to be courageous leadership through the neutral zone to allow new ways of working to become established. Then, and only then, can there be a genuinely new beginning. Too often, such changes are attempted without sufficient appreciation of the transition process required and then abandoned without the lessons being learned.

Clarity of purpose plays an important part in enabling a new beginning. Everyone involved, not just the top team, needs to grasp the reason for change and the benefits it will bring. From the boardroom to the reception desk, there should be a clear understanding of what is changing, why it has to change and what will be gained. Often in organisations you will overhear conversations which go along the lines of:

> *Supervisor*: 'From now on we'll be ordering supplies using this system.'
> *Employee*: 'It looks complicated. Why can't we stick with the old system?'
> *Supervisor*: 'Don't ask me. I'm just passing on what I've been told.'

Such an exchange ought to ring alarm bells. Once the purpose of the change has been lost, the best that can now be achieved is grudging compliance. But the answer does not lie in doubling the number of briefing sessions. The best way to connect people to the purpose of change is to involve them in the change process. But even if the change is inevitable and local management has little or no influence over its implementation, explaining the reasons for a new system or procedure – particularly ones that link it to improved patient care – will help staff adapt. In the throes of a protracted change project it is easy to lose sight of purpose, but it's important to make sure that staff are aware of the improvements their efforts will create.

Vision is a step beyond purpose. Whereas purpose supplies the reason for the inconvenience and uncertainty staff must put up with, vision paints a compelling picture of how things will be. For many of us, mere facts do not fire the imagination and we need something more to engage our enthusiasm. Seeing what something is like plays a huge part in decision making, a fact well understood by the advertising industry. When we buy a car, it is not enough to know the performance specifications, we want to know what it looks like. That's why, in car advertisements, the picture takes up most of the space and the technical details are in tiny print at the bottom of the page. When an architect wants to sell us a design for a building, he doesn't just tell us the dimensions of the rooms and the materials he would employ. Instead, he tries to convey the experience of actually living in the design by using drawings and models. A vision in change management works in a similar way, giving staff a vivid impression of what it will be like to work with the new system or new equipment. You may need to use your imagination as to how this can be done.

➤ One hospital, going through the process of moving staff and patients from an institutional to a community-based service, got staff to visualise and then write down a day in the life of one of their patients in the new setting. The exercise proved to be a turning point in the attitudes of the staff involved. Although the purpose and plans had already been explained to them, they now 'saw' what it would really be like and the freedom it would give to their patients.

➤ If the change you are working towards is already up and running somewhere else, why not organise a visit so people can see what it looks like in action. This will be more persuasive and informative than a dozen presentations or reports.

Change is holistic

Here are two mini case studies based on real life.

➤ A hospital facing financial problems decided to severely limit the ability of managers to buy in nursing staff from agencies to cover shortages. This was a perfectly understandable response to a serious issue and savings were duly made. Some weeks later, managers noticed a growing number of complaints about junior staff being left in charge of hospital wards. This was dealt with as a new problem but, on reflection, it was a direct result of the action taken to solve the earlier problem.

➤ To avoid patients waiting long periods of time for treatment, a target of four hours was set for emergency patients arriving at English NHS hospitals to be either discharged or admitted. This had the unexpected consequence of increasing emergency admissions as hospitals set up special wards to admit patients who would take longer than four hours to diagnose and treat.[16] Another unintended consequence were the reports of patients being kept waiting in ambulances to avoid letting them into hospital and thus starting the clock running on the target.

What these examples illustrate is that when we introduce change into one part of an organisation, the consequences will be felt in other parts or in unexpected ways.

A little like when we press down on an airbed and the pressure we exert on one part causes another part to rise. Because organisations are an interconnected network of people and resources, changes ripple out across the whole system. The consequences may be delayed, may be positive or negative, or they may be felt in an entirely different area but there will be consequences. Peter Senge calls this 'the classic dilemma of problem solving in complex systems. We don't see the larger structures within which we are operating. Consequently our actions come back to haunt us – or to haunt someone else, someone in another part of the system or someone in the future'.[17] If we see problems in isolation, our attempts to fix them may create even bigger problems. This law of unintended consequences applies to any complex living system, such as an ecosystem or even the human body.

This is similar to iatrogenic (doctor-caused) illness where patients experience health problems as a direct result of the treatment of another illness. Although the intention was good, the unforeseen consequence is negative. Sometimes the cause of the problem is polypharmacy – the combination of drugs being taken by the patient. Each drug may have been correctly prescribed for a particular condition but because the body is a connected whole, not a collection of separate parts, the cumulative effect is illness rather than health. In the same way, organisations can suffer from manager-caused illness as various change initiatives, all of which make perfect sense when considered in isolation, combine to induce change fatigue with its symptoms of cynicism and mistrust.

Whole-systems thinking

The lesson we must draw from all of this is that we must think about change in its wider context. One perspective on a situation and what needs to be done is unlikely to be enough. The other people or agencies involved need to be part of the process of thinking through the issue and generating a solution. This means much more than consultation, where people are asked to respond to a limited set of predetermined options. We need to allow those directly involved in the issue to contribute, from their different perspectives, to a collaborative improvement process. Depending on the issue, this may mean a whole team or a whole workforce. Participation may need to include several professions or even several organisations. Done well, this reduces the risk of unintended consequences and turns implementation from an adversarial test of strength to a shared journey.

People can change themselves

We don't believe that people don't like change. If this were true, house moves, holidays, marriages and promotions would be rare. We would argue that what most people don't like is *being* changed, where they are forced to adapt to choices made by other people. So if people feel that they have some influence over organisational change, they are less likely to want to oppose or sabotage it. Just as importantly, by giving people the opportunity to be involved, we enable them to bring their creativity and insight to bear on the problem. Command and control management by a senior team not only creates resistance, it also ignores the contribution that could have been made by staff who are closer to the issues being addressed.

Whilst senior managers are often best placed to define and clarify the problems that face a department or organisation and to set the ground rules for change, they are not well placed to dictate detailed solutions. Their best contribution is to skilfully manage a process which enables staff to collaborate in identifying and implementing improvements within their own work areas. For this to happen, staff must be liberated from micro-management and excessive controls. And this does not just apply at times of major change. Many organisations are moving towards much greater empowerment of their staff, giving them more access to and control over resources and information. Instead of decisions frequently having to be passed up the hierarchy for resolution, teams who work closest to the customer or patient solve problems for themselves. Not only is this quicker, it also means that decisions are better informed and more sensitive to the needs of each unique situation. One of the major barriers in establishing these empowered or self-directed teams is the mindset of managers who equate management with control and who see the empowerment of their staff as threatening.

WHEN MANAGEMENT CONTROL MAKES THINGS WORSE:
AN EXAMPLE FROM CHILD PROTECTION

In 2010, in the wake of several well-publicised scandals involving child abuse, the UK government asked Professor Eileen Munro to review arrangements for child protection. She found that targets and procedures were emphasised to such an extent that they had taken the focus of professionals away from the very children they were employed to protect. The review recommended 'a radical reduction in the amount of central prescription to help professionals move from a compliance culture to a learning culture'.[18] Using a systems approach, Professor Munro identified the unintended consequences of excessive control. Having too many procedures limits the scope of professional judgement, which leads to a reduction in job satisfaction and self-esteem, which in turn leads to increased sickness and absence. The consequence of this is larger caseloads and therefore less time for professionals to build relationships with children and families. This inevitably reduces the quality of outcomes, which further reduces job satisfaction. This becomes a vicious circle where the negative effects of too many controls increase over time, even though the original intention of the rules and procedures was to improve care.

At times of change, especially when things are not going the way we hoped, it is tempting to see more controls as the answer. But perversely, as the example above illustrates, overcontrol of staff can actually cause the problems that the controls were designed to eliminate. Perhaps management control in organisations is like salt in flavouring meals. While just a little is good, this doesn't mean that more will be better. After all, taken in sufficient quantities, salt is an emetic. Likewise, when it comes to change and innovation, increasing control is almost always not the answer. Too much leads to a sick organisation.

The idea that change has to be led or influenced, rather than controlled, makes many managers nervous. If true, much has to be unlearned and a new set of skills developed. To constructively involve people in the process of change is much more testing than simply giving orders. To develop teams that will take the initiative to solve their own problems requires the questioning of principles that many managers see as foundational. Skills in listening and facilitation are required and, even more challenging, the hope, courage and humility that go with good leadership. Instead of controlling, auditing and problem solving, leaders of empowered teams have to turn their attention to developing the team and making sure it has the skills, resources and systems to become self-managing. This is hard for managers whose personal fulfilment comes from a sense of being needed 24 hours a day.

These managers need careful preparation to be able to embrace the idea that their staff might actually do better without their minute-by-minute intervention and constant checking. Faced with these mountains to climb, some might retreat to the familiar territory of command and control management. After all, it is easier, quicker and so widely utilised that no one is likely to be criticised for managing in this way. But to do so flies in the face of the evidence. If what we want is innovation and lasting improvement, command and control are ineffective. Even if we dress it up with consultations, toolkits and roll-outs, change imposed inflexibly by the few upon the many fails more often than it works. Given the opportunity, staff can introduce change themselves.

INFLUENCING CHANGE: THE NEW PRINCIPLES

Our recognition of the inadequacies of top-down change and the need to treat people as humans rather than components must, if it is to mean anything, be translated into a new approach to change. The principles set out below are a way of putting into practice our acknowledgement that change is a people issue, not just a technical one; that change is a process not an event; that change is holistic and that people can change themselves

This is not a step-by-step checklist, where actions can be ticked off when completed. The principles below need to guide our influencing at every stage.

➤ Connect people to purpose.

➤ Clarify and maintain focus.

➤ Clarify targets, and any boundaries and non-negotiables.

➤ Involve people constructively.

➤ Positive accountability.

Connect people to purpose

The idea of 'vocation' may be not a particularly fashionable one but finding meaning in our work is a powerful motivating force. In influencing change, we need to work with this force, connecting the change with what is important to the people involved. Michael Fullan, who has successfully influenced change in education systems in the USA, UK and Canada, calls this the 'moral purpose'.[19] He found that where teachers came to believe that the purpose of a new initiative was to improve the life chances of young people, they treated it seriously rather than cynically. This means more than making a glib statement at the start of the process. The moral purpose must be something that activates and shapes the whole change programme or people will realise that it was never genuine. Fullan stresses the importance of moral purpose and the high expectations that flow from it. After all, if we really are talking about quality of life and the well-being of a community, we must aim high.

Most NHS staff are motivated by providing excellent care for patients[20] and this desire is a positive force for change. Being able to demonstrate a clear connection between what we are asking staff to do and the health of patients enables us to harness this desire. If no such connection is made we can confidently expect people to see what we are doing as no more than change for change's sake.

So what is the moral purpose that drives the change you want to see? How will it benefit patients and how will you know it has worked? If not only you but your team can answer this with confidence, you will be well on the way to willing commitment, not grudging compliance.

Clarify and maintain focus

We have tried to show that the manager cannot control change and that attempting to micro-manage people will, in the end, be counterproductive. But this doesn't mean that managers have no role in change. If we want people to commit to innovation and improvement, we have to show our own commitment by maintaining our focus and not losing interest or launching other disconnected or even conflicting programmes. This will require self-discipline and courage, particularly when senior colleagues want to show their leadership by announcing another change programme. This is often the result of a knee-jerk reaction to a problem or perhaps just impatience (see the section on 'something must be done!' in Chapter 1). For staff to be able to collaborate in improving the service, managers must clarify the overall direction of travel and set out any non-negotiables. Having done this, the focus needs to be maintained relentlessly. Depending on the scale of the change, this relentless focus may need to be sustained for months or even years.

CHANGE FATIGUE

One of us, many years ago, was given the task of writing and promoting a new national management development strategy for the Welsh health service. Unaware of the own-goals he had already scored by trying to tell thousands of people, in detail, what to do, he planned a tour of chief executives to promote the new strategy document. To this day, he remembers the look of weariness on the face of one top manager who produced a stack of other documents – all recent initiatives – that he was also being asked to embrace with enthusiasm. Change fatigue had set in.

Clarify targets, and any boundaries or non-negotiables

If we want staff to play a part in bringing about change, they have to know what they are aiming for and what limits, e.g. money or time, apply. To use a sports analogy, players need to know the rules of the game and they need to be able to clearly see the markings on the pitch. Once these are clarified, they can use their own skills and ingenuity to get a result.

Involving staff in change does not mean that they have complete freedom, and most are smart enough to understand this. They know that there will always be constraints, such as the need to stay within budget or maintain a certain level of service. Constraints may also be imposed by legislation or professional codes of practice. Early in the change process, the boundaries and non-negotiables need to be made abundantly clear, and even if you wish there was more room for manoeuvre, it is best to be honest. Giving staff the impression that they have more freedom than is really the case will be counterproductive when, further down the line, they have to be told that some of their ideas are impractical because of previously undeclared constraints. Enthusiasm and trust will inevitably be damaged as they realise that critical information was withheld. We have observed the disastrous effect on morale when staff are asked to join in with a process of consultation or engagement only to find that the outcome was a foregone conclusion.

So, the rules – the non-negotiables – need to declared. But, and it's a big but, there should be as few rules as possible. This is sometimes called a loose-tight approach, where the rules are firm but few, leaving lots of room for innovation. Too many rules, and people will understand that they are not really being trusted.

Involve people constructively

For this to happen, there must be a genuine recognition of the inadequacy of top-down change and a conviction that involving people is not merely a gesture but the way to release innovation and achieve sustainability. In many organisations, top management often attempt to involve staff through consultation meetings. These normally take the form of presentations from the front, plus time for questions. The format of the meeting and even the layout of the room, where people sit in rows facing a stage, reinforce the idea that what people should do is shut up and listen. As a result, little in the way of meaningful discussion happens and staff go away frustrated that they have not really been heard. Such meetings may do more harm than good but they continue to be held, partly through laziness and partly because alternative methods of involvement are not known or understood.

➤ **Involve from the start**. If you are consulting on your ideas for change, you are already leaving involvement too late. You needn't be the one who comes up with the solutions, you just have to make sure a solution is found. Gather the staff involved and outline how you see the problem. Let them know about any constraints or non-negotiables and let them join you in identifying possible ways forward. Instead of sitting them in rows, seat them around tables to promote discussion. Ask them to feed back their ideas and listen carefully. Use skilled facilitators to make sure the process is constructive and participative or employ a technique such as 'World Café'[21] that provides a simple structure which allows large numbers of people to collaborate in putting forward ideas and proposals (see box).

WORLD CAFÉ: A TECHNIQUE FOR INVOLVEMENT AND OWNERSHIP

World Café brings together groups of people to generate ideas, share knowledge and discover opportunities for practical action. Participants sit around tables instead of in rows and instead of a leader or tutor, there is a host who gets the ball rolling by setting an open question such as 'what would make the biggest difference to our patients?' or 'what would bring about change on this issue?'. The groups discuss the question and note down, usually on the paper tablecloth, key ideas or themes. After 30 minutes, all but one of the people on each table disperse to other tables and work on another question designed to move the discussion on. The person who remains tells the next set of people at the table the main points from the previous dialogue and they carry on from there, adding their words and drawings to those already on the tablecloth.

Most World Café events would have three rounds of progressive dialogue after which there is a whole-group discussion to reflect on what has been learned. With thoughtful hosting, World Café usually leads to the emergence of themes, ideas or possibilities for action that are widely shared and owned.

➤ **Involve widely**. Don't assume that only senior professionals should have a voice. Junior or untrained staff and service users can bring valuable ideas and insights. If the changes will affect other organisations or departments, invite them to be part of the process. The general rule is, if they are affected, they should be involved.

➤ **Encourage peer networking**. People listen to their peers. In fact, person-to-person influencing in the context of social networks has been found to be the 'dominant mechanism for promoting adoption of innovations'.[22] Such networks needn't be expensive or cumbersome, and the rewards can be significant, so the wise organisation will actively encourage its professional staff to network widely.

➤ **Involve constructively**. Having set the direction of travel and clarified the targets or boundaries, managers need to enable staff to get involved practically. One technique which has proved successful in healthcare organisations is PDSA, or plan, do, study, act, which allows staff to collaborate in order to solve problems or make improvements. A 'hands on, fingers out' approach is required whereby management trains staff in PDSA and actively encourages and supports, but does not micro-manage. The essence of PDSA is that small changes are made and then evaluated, refined and tested again. This cycle continues, with staff working on a small scale before larger changes are made. In complex systems like healthcare organisations, this step-by-step approach is far safer than the 'big bang' variety of change. It also allows change to be initiated in many places within the organisation, driven by the staff who actually provide the service. The role of senior management in this is to equip, support and relentlessly maintain direction and focus.

PDSA CASE STUDY: SETTING UP A DISCHARGE LOUNGE

A hospital wanted to avoid the problem of patients waiting for a bed whose occupant had been medically discharged but whose transport had not yet arrived. After analysing patient throughput data, they decided to use PDSA to investigate the potential value of a discharge lounge.

Plan A proposal for a temporary discharge lounge was drawn up, including a protocol for how it would operate, the facilities it would need and the staff required.

Do The hospital arranged to use school facilities on the hospital site over a three-day half-term period when it was not in use. Bed managers and wards were briefed along with other linked departments such as pharmacy. A welcome desk and entertainment facilities for patients and carers were also organised.

Study All throughput times were carefully measured over the three days. Several clear advantages were found.

- ➤ No patient breached the 4-hour waiting target
- ➤ Beds were freed up earlier
- ➤ Improved patient satisfaction
- ➤ An opportunity for reverse usage for elective patients coming in
- ➤ Lighter nursing load

But several areas for improvement were also identified such as the design of the area and the absence of seating for special needs patients.

Act On the basis of the test, a longer test was scheduled with improvements made to the original design. This test revealed that the lounge was mainly used by patients waiting for take-home drugs, which highlighted another opportunity for improvement. This longer test provided even better data on which to assess the value of a discharge lounge.

Adapted from Walley P, Gowland B. Completing the circle: from PD to PDSA. *Int J Health Care Qual Assur.* 2004; **17**(6): 349–58.

Positive accountability

How will you judge that progress is being made? Like the non-negotiables, there need to be a few, clear targets so that progress can be measured. This might be the number of patients treated, a reduction in infection rates or waiting times, or an increase in patient satisfaction. The targets and data on progress need to be open and transparent so that everyone involved has feedback on their efforts and can see how they are doing in comparison with others. Healthy rivalry and pride in achievement are strong motivators. Progress should be rewarded, celebrated and shared so that good ideas can spread around peer networks. As a last resort, in the case of a lack of progress, the triggers for active intervention need to be clear. But the focus here is on rewarding and encouraging, not punishing.

STARTING SMALL: CREATIVE CONVERSATIONS

These five principles provide a way of influencing change founded on the need to liberate the creativity and energy of the people who work in healthcare organisations. We offer them as a realistic alternative to the top-down change which is so often operationally ineffective and destructive of morale. Whether you sit at the top of an organisation or at grass roots, we hope you will agree that change cannot really be controlled, only led or influenced. For this reason, even if you have no formal authority to implement change, we would suggest that much of what we have put forward still holds good. Even without a top management position, there is no reason why you cannot engage people in creative conversations about the way things are and the way they might be. Indeed, some would say that change can be seen not as the technical task of implementing plans but as 'a living craft'[23] of participating in small-scale conversations and encounters with people which reshape our thinking and, therefore, the future.

If you see the need for change in departments or agencies where you have no formal power, why not initiate a conversation? Not to sell an idea or to overwhelm people with your logic, but simply to explore together how things might be different. Where an aggressive attempt to persuade might provoke defensiveness, a genuine invitation to think things through together will appeal to the innate curiosity of many. You could do this informally or you could initiate a 'World Café' style event, perhaps in a local coffee house, where anyone with an interest could come to exchange ideas about how the service or organisation could be improved. And if you are wondering whether you are allowed to do this, it may be helpful to remember that it is sometimes better to ask for forgiveness than permission!

To work in this grass-roots, collaborative way means that your contribution may go unrecognised. But if you can bear to be the facilitator rather than the architect of change, much can be achieved by bringing people together to think, hope and dream.

LEARNING FROM EXPERIENCE

Think about changes you have recently instigated or helped to introduce. These could be changes in work patterns, procedures, structures or the physical layout of the workplace.

How successfully was the change introduced and how, in the light of this chapter, do you account for this?

To what extent, and in what way, were people constructively involved?

What do you think you most need to do differently next time?

RECOMMENDED READING

➤ To understand change as a process, we recommend *Managing Transitions* by William Bridges, published by Nicholas Brealey, or *The Challenge of Change in Organisations* by Nancy Barger and Linda Kirby, published by Davies-Black.

➤ For guidance on how to lead change in a complex organisation, try *Leading in a Culture of Change* by Michael Fullan, published by Jossey-Bass. Although Fullan writes about education, the lessons are transferable.

➤ For practical ways to involve people in change, try *The World Café* by Juanita Brown or *Terms of Engagement* by Richard Axelrod, both published by Berrett-Koehler.

➤ To find out more about empowered teams, we recommend *Leading Self-Directed Work Teams* by Kimball Fisher, published by McGraw-Hill.

REFERENCES

1 Axelrod R. *Terms of Engagement*. San Francisco: Berrett-Koehler; 2010.
2 Palmer I, Hardy C. *Thinking about Management*. London: Sage; 2000. p.192.
3 Wheatley M. *Leadership and the New Science*. San Francisco: Berrett-Koehler: 1999. p.138.
4 IBM Corporation. *Making Change Work*. Somers, NY: IBM Corporation; 2008. www-935.ibm.com/services/us/gbs/bus/html/gbs-making-change-work.html
5 Chartered Institute for Personnel and Development. *Reorganising for Success: CEOs' and HR managers' perceptions*. London: Chartered Institute for Personnel and Development; 2003. p.36.
6 Olson E, Eoyang E. *Facilitating Organization Change*. San Francisco: Jossey-Bass; 2001. p.3.
7 Sheldrake J. *Management Theory*. 2nd ed. London: Thomson; 2003.
8 Higgs MJ, Rowland D. Change and its leadership: is it time for a change in our thinking? *Proceedings of the ECLO Conference*, Prague, 2006.
9 Taylor FW. *The Principles of Scientific Management*. New York: Harper and Row; 1911.
10 Hamel G. *The Future of Management*. Boston: Harvard Business Press; 2007. p.255.
11 Price Waterhouse Coopers. Innovation Survey. 1999. p.3. www.wowgreatidea.com/articles/7_PWCInnovationSurvey.pdf. In a 1999 survey of companies in the *Financial Times* 100, Price Waterhouse Coopers found that the most significant factor differentiating successful from unsuccessful innovators was management trust. 'The top performers empowered individuals to communicate and implement change...'
12 Finlayson B. *Counting the Smiles: morale and motivation in the NHS*. London: King's Fund; 2002. Research by the King's Fund found that, for NHS staff, the most significant determinant of motivation in the workplace was the extent to which they felt valued. www.kingsfund.org.uk/publications/counting_the.html
13 Sarros J, Cooper B, Santora J. Building a climate for innovation through transformation leadership and organisational culture. *J Leadership Organiz Studies*. 2008. www.allbusiness.com/company-activities-management/management-corporate-culture/11674769-1.html A survey of 1158 managers found that a leadership style which articulated a vision was strongly associated with innovative organisations.

Other significant leadership behaviours were supporting employees and having high expectations of them.

14 Bridges W. *Managing Transitions*. 2nd ed. London: Nicholas Brealey, 2003.

15 Kübler-Ross E. *On Death and Dying*. London: Routledge; 1969.

16 Robinson P. Data Briefing. *Health Service J.* 2007; **October**. www.chks.co.uk/assets/files/DataBriefings/A&E_4hr_tgt_HSJ18Oct07.pdf

17 Senge P. Lecture at the Annual Conference of the Robert K Greenleaf Centre, October 1992. Cited in: Spears L, editor. *Reflections on Leadership*. New York: Wiley; 1995.

18 Department for Education. *The Munro Review of Child Protection: Final Report*. Cm 8062. London: Department for Education; 2011. p.7.

19 Fullan M. *All Systems Go*. Thousand Oaks: Corwin; 2010. p.62.

20 Ipsos MORI. *What Matters to Staff in the NHS*. Research conducted for the Department of Health. London: Department of Health; 2008.

21 Brown J. *The World Café: shaping our future through conversations that matter*. San Francisco: Berrett-Koehler; 2005.

22 Greenhalgh T, Robert G, Bate P, Kyriakidou O, Macfarlane F, Peacock R. *How to Spread Good Ideas*. London: National Co-ordinating Centre for NHS Service Delivery and Organisation; 2004. p.17.

23 Shaw P. *Changing Conversations in Organisations*. London: Routledge; 2002. p.172.

CHAPTER 5

Influencing in formal settings

Throughout your management and influencing career there will be times when opportunities present themselves 'in the moment' and have to be grasped. To balance this, there will also be times when your influencing will take place in a formalised, and often choreographed, environment such as an official meeting or a negotiation. This chapter offers a range of quite precise and technical approaches to help you influence in these situations.

Typically those formal settings will have the following characteristics.

➤ A prearranged date and time.

➤ A formal environment such as a boardroom, conference centre venue, or a senior manager's office.

➤ Two or more parties or interests represented 'at the table'.

➤ The meeting is a result of one or more of the following:

  – an actual failure to resolve an issue in previous, more informal settings

  – a perception by one or more parties that the issue is best dealt with formally from the start

  – a history of such issues being subject to formal negotiation

  – the need for 'due process' to be seen and recorded (particularly prevalent in Apollo cultures – see Chapter 3).

➤ The need for a level of emotional detachment, even if the issues being discussed affect you and your team personally and deeply.

Please note that this chapter does not advocate the stereotypical caricature of hostile, fist-thumping protagonists on opposite sides of the table, each having introduced patently outrageous starting positions and who are intent on playing mind games, in pursuit of the opportunity to showboat to their constituents.

In healthcare settings the emphasis throughout needs to be professional, collaborative where possible, and mindful of the need to work together after the negotiating episode is concluded. In short, it requires both maturity and a mutual desire to confine any disagreement to the issues, not the individuals.

The subtext for this book is influencing *with integrity* and we firmly believe that, whilst staff in the same organisation can and should sometimes have robust and strong-willed negotiations, there is no long-term benefit in outflanking or humiliating the very colleagues you will have to work with in the future. Therefore this chapter is all about conducting yourself in a professional, committed but always reasonable manner, whilst still seeking to influence the other parties into action that benefits your team or service.

YOU KNOW MORE THAN YOU THINK!

We are sometimes asked by our health service clients to deliver programmes on 'negotiation skills'. Given that many of the delegates on such courses would be experienced clinicians, it is quite likely that they will already be experts! When a nurse works with a challenging patient or a demanding set of relatives, they are employing quite sophisticated negotiation skills. When a family doctor helps an obese or substance-misusing patient through a change of lifestyle, they will be constantly looking for the levers of influence and bringing in additional arguments as new barriers emerge. When a multidisciplinary ward team is discussing an imminent discharge, the occupational therapist is often engaged in a three-way negotiation involving the local authority and the community services responsible for care in the home environment.

Therefore we start this chapter by asking readers to access and use their own skills of influencing and negotiating, rather than leave them at the door and assume that formal influencing settings involve some sort of dark art. Yes, the setting is different, and yes, the choreography can be a little stilted to start with, but the basics are still there.

➤ All parties must have a legitimate interest in the issue.

➤ Those who would like to see change must have a credible proposal.

➤ Those involved must have either the direct authority to approve or veto any agreement, or timely access to that authority.

➤ One of the parties has something that the other needs (money, staff, approval, endorsement, expertise, etc.) which cannot or should not be obtained by means of status or force.

➤ The behaviour of those involved will be, in part, influenced by personalities, organisational cultures, history, and the way others communicate with them.

A USEFUL DEFINITION OF NEGOTIATION?

A **process**, triggered by a **problem or proposal**, in which **two or more parties bargain** over a **range of issues** with the intention of reaching a **mutually beneficial agreement**.

This definition has been deliberately constructed to include a number of important features.

➤ It is a *process*, not an event, and complex negotiations may take place over an extended time period.

➤ The existing situation is likely to be unsatisfactory (at least to one of the parties), otherwise why is everyone there?

➤ There may often be more than two parties involved in the process – don't assume it is always two. Indeed, having more than two parties can add more opportunities for finding solutions although it can make the process a little more complex.

➤ There can often be more than one connected issue 'on the table', and multiplicity can actually provide flexibility at the bargaining stage.

➤ Bargaining assumes that the parties involved are mandated to do so and can make binding agreements.

➤ Mutually beneficial means just that – all parties need to be able to take something positive away otherwise the process will lack respect.

It is important to point out that if you are going into any formal negotiating situation with complete authority to demand one, and only one, acceptable outcome, and you have absolutely no flexibility and nothing to offer in return, please don't call it negotiation. It is simply giving an instruction and demanding compliance!

A better approach is to assume that all parties need to be able to answer the simple **WIIFM** question – What's In It For Me? – where 'me' is shorthand for my team/organisation/constituency/profession, etc. Unless there can be a positive answer to that question for each party, why should they bother to turn up?

Whilst we are on the subject of power and authority, step back a moment and ask yourself: 'Where does the power come from when I do my job?'. In other words, how do you manage to get things done by others? Whilst there are many sources of power, five common ones are shown in the table opposite. You will often use a combination of these but, just as we have personality and cultural default preferences, we tend to fall back on one or two of these power sources, particularly when under pressure.

All of these sources of power can and should be brought to bear in the formal negotiation process, but do some thinking first. Useful questions to ask before you enter the negotiation arena include the following.

➤ How do I tend to come across and will that be helpful in this situation?

➤ Who else will be there and how might they approach the process?

➤ Are there others in my team whose personal style might be more appropriate, either to lead the process or to assist me in dealing with certain people?

Source	Manifestation	Useful for	Potential pitfalls
Technical expertise	Having and demonstrating a firm grasp of the relevant subject	Reassurance and confidence building, particularly in situations where the risks of failure are seen to be high	Can come across as know it all, or even condescending when dealing with those outside your professional area
Positional authority	The power that comes from your hierarchical position, regardless of your intrinsic knowledge or ability	Being clear on any non-negotiables on behalf of your organisation, and for demonstrating the ability to commit to the final decision	Can be seen as an easy fallback position when you are losing the argument
Charisma and personality	Your sheer enthusiasm or excitement that infects others	Raising spirits, building commitment and motivation, and inspiring others	Can be seen by others as naivety or enthusiasm designed to mask the real problems
Winning hearts and minds	Appealing to people's values, higher purpose and intrinsic motivation	Connecting the issues being discussed to core purpose, reminding people of the bigger picture	Can come across as a little preachy (as if you are trying to impose your values on others)
Laid back, 'laissez faire'	Appearing to simply set out the issue and not take an obvious position either positive or negative	Allowing the merits of a case to speak for themselves and not being seen to challenge others' position or authority	Can be seen as uninterested and lacking in personal drive

The purpose of these questions is not to build some kind of 'shock and awe' dream team, or to completely neutralise the legitimate behaviours of the other parties. You are simply trying to ensure that the process is constructive and productive. You may have heard media reports of negotiations breaking down at the 11th hour amid rancour and militant talk, and at one level we are fascinated by such stories. However, they are not pleasant to be part of, and anything you can do to keep the process going with professionalism and dignity will be rewarded in the long run. Remember our earlier statement that you have to work with these people afterwards, so make sure any disagreement stays with the issues, not the people.

What those questions should do is make you stop and think about who is best placed to carry out the negotiations, given the issues, the people and the history. Some of the best influencing you will ever do will be achieved by stepping aside and letting others lead the way.

THE PROCESS OF FORMAL NEGOTIATION

Once you are clear who needs to be involved and why, you can look at the formal process.

This does tend to follow a standard framework, but it is vital that you see it as just that – a framework, not a cage. All parties need to be able to customise the process to fit the time available, the nature of the issues, the prior history and relationships between the parties, and the way the dialogue develops on a given day. However, it is useful to have a broad framework as this can help to reintroduce a neutral process if and when the conversation loses focus or gets heated.

Stage	Tasks, questions and behaviour
Preparation	• Think through your issue carefully – why is it a problem, what is needed, and what consequences might there be? • Would a document help to set the scene? If so, in what style and detail? • What are the legitimate interests of the other parties? In their shoes, how would you respond to the proposal or problem? • Behave in a mature manner, and set up the process with care and dignity. Don't allow your frustration to leak out in any correspondence or conversations at this stage as this could set the wrong tone. • Find out how the other parties would prefer to handle the negotiation process and, where possible, build those wishes into the final structure.
Plan your strategy	• Assuming you are the proactive party (you are instigating the process in pursuit of your objectives), how will you handle the first negotiating session? • How will you lay out the room? It is worth bearing in mind that hostile argument is less likely if the protagonists are sitting next to each other (and more likely when facing each other across a table!). • If you are negotiating as part of a duo or larger team, you are advised to separate the chairing role from the presenting/arguing role to prevent perceptions of using procedure to favour your case. • It is a good idea to plan to start the meeting with quick 'round the table' statements of what people are hoping to get from the session today – this gives you clues as to their level of engagement, degree of decision-making power, and any areas of concern. It also confirms the chair's role in managing the process.
Present your proposal	• What will you include in your presentation? Understanding the cultures and personalities of the other parties will give you good clues as to the best approach. If in doubt, be crisp, factual, brief and professional without being slick or condescending. • Recognise that you will have been living and breathing this issue for some time – possibly months – but the other parties may be hearing it in detail for the first time. Therefore don't overload the presentation and don't get carried away with emotion. People don't like being preached to!

Stage	Tasks, questions and behaviour
Listen	• The one mouth/two ears principle comes into play here. Once you have presented, shut up and genuinely listen to the responses. Avoid at all costs the urge to fix or undermine each point or objection as it comes up. At this stage simply acknowledge them as genuine and worthy of respect. • In some scenarios, the other parties will want to make their own presentation, either introducing new ideas or challenging your proposals. Give them the same courtesy you demanded from them, then state any objections in a calm manner and don't expect them to be answered immediately.
Engage in true *dialogue*	• In this context, dialogue means a collaborative exchange aimed at a joint solution. Contrast this with debate (which means to beat down) or discussion (which has the same root word as percussion). • Dialogue involves honouring the contributions of others and looking for ways of building on those ideas, as opposed to always looking to knock the other ideas away and replace them with your own. It can be a powerful tool in the bargaining process and helps all parties to walk away with something to sell to their constituents.
Bargain	• This is the stage most closely related to our common perceptions of negotiation. Some call it horse trading, haggling or bartering, but it is potentially the least dignified part of the process. For this reason it is often the most secretive element and is rarely talked about in press conferences afterwards! • At its most basic, this is the *quid pro quo* stuff of 'If you do this, I will do that' or 'We will accept less than we asked for if you will bring forward your plans for X'. • Clearly this will only work if you do have some degree of flexibility, and you do need to have agreed any 'wriggle room' with your colleagues in advance. • If, during this period of offer and counteroffer, you are surprised by a particular contribution or feel that the whole thing is getting out of control, use the *adjournment* approach. This might be for just a few minutes or it could be until the next planned session, but it can really help to calm things down, allow mature reflection on the various contributions, and ensure that your own concessions are sustainable.
Agree	• Negotiations often go on longer than necessary because of a failure to capture and then protect agreements as they emerge. The chair's role is vital in this respect and their ability to summarise and seek agreement is a critical part of the process. • There are three types of agreement the chair should be watching out for. 1 Agreement about the existence and severity of the **problem** (you cannot hope to get agreement on a solution until this stage has been reached). 2 Agreement on one or more of the **ideas** being put forward (look for emerging areas of agreement and log these to prevent them being unpicked later). 3 Agreement on where the parties continue to **disagree**, and the actions to resolve these areas (don't leave loose ends – make sure every point, however contentious, has some clear outcome, even if it is just further research to clarify the disputed facts).

DEALING WITH UNHELPFUL BEHAVIOUR

Despite the mature and reasonable approach advocated above, there will be times when human beings become unreasonable. Typical behaviours, and some suggested responses, are given below.

Behaviour	Suggested response
Making threats – warning of unwelcome repercussions	Make it clear that there will be no negotiations under duress.
Offering insults	Stay calm, restate your position, acknowledge the reasonable concerns of the other parties, but introduce the possibility of breaking off and reconvening on another day if not more constructive.
Bluff – threats of non-specific consequences	Call their bluff – calmly ask for the evidence and suggest that, if the tables were turned, this threatening approach to the negotiations would not be appreciated by the other parties.
Divide and rule, whereby a statement by one of you is compared unfavourably with a statement by another team member	Brief team in advance on how contributions will be given and by whom – call an adjournment if you feel the team is losing focus or cutting across another team member's area.
Asking leading questions	Don't answer – or attach conditions to your reply.
Emotional appeals	Restate issues calmly – don't join in with the 'my emotional appeal beats your emotional appeal' game.

HINTS AND TIPS FOR NEGOTIATING IN TEAMS

➤ Ensure all team members have a value in being there. Going in as a gang will be seen as a clumsy attempt to intimidate and is more likely to lead to antagonism and suspicion. Make it clear from the start who is there, why they are there, and then stick rigidly to those roles.

➤ Be clear who is the lead negotiator and let them do most of the talking. As soon as the other parties see different people chipping in, they will see an opportunity to exploit inconsistencies. Once someone has said 'That's interesting but it is different from what your colleague said earlier', you are on the back foot and the other side is bound to play on whichever statement was the most favourable to their argument.

➤ The lead negotiator must bring in the other players and their expertise as he or she thinks necessary. Do not interrupt or correct your own team members.

➤ If a silent team member is uneasy at the way things are progressing, call for a short adjournment. Agree beforehand some system for alerting the lead negotiator as passing hastily scribbled notes up the table looks unprofessional and may give the other parties an unwarranted advantage.

SUMMARY

We hope that the core message communicated in this highly practical chapter is that the atmosphere in which formal negotiations are carried out can be as influential as the case or arguments being put forward. When you are entering negotiations with colleagues and peers from within your own organisation, this becomes even more important given that you will have to deal with those people again and again in the future.

We would argue that one of the most valuable things you can develop in your career is a reputation – in this case a reputation as someone whom others can do business with. That is not management speak for a soft touch, simply an acknowledgement that, whilst you may disagree on the case or proposal, you can still build a reputation as someone who acts honourably. Not only will this reputation help with any current negotiations, it will increase the chances of success next time, regardless of the outcome this time.

In contrast, if you gather a reputation for petulant behaviour, underhand methods and reacting inappropriately to either success and failure, your ability to influence others will rapidly decline.

It is worth stressing that no amount of good negotiation practice will rescue a poor proposal. Conversely, good proposals are often harmed by weak, or overbearing, negotiation strategies. You will not win your case every time. Why? Because organisations are made up of people, not machines, and logic will not always win the day. However, if you approach the whole task with integrity and good faith, the chances of continued success are considerably improved.

As one of us was told some years ago, even though we had had robust disagreements with the person over the years: 'You are someone I can do business with'.

We advise you to build the same reputation, by improving the way you handle the challenging and sometimes stilted atmosphere of formal influencing settings. In contrast to the team leader who develops a reputation for 'taking on' opponents on behalf of their team (amusing in the short term but ultimately embarrassing to everyone), your team will thank you for your professionalism and indeed will share in your deserved reputation.

CHAPTER 6

Being a role model

The greatest influencing tool or resource at your disposal is **you**. So, having looked at some of the external factors in influencing – such as organisational culture, change methods, formal tactics, etc. – we now return to how your own approach can either help or hinder your success. This chapter will have a far more technical 'toolkit' feel to it, as we offer you a menu of processes and methods that, individually or in tandem, will increase your personal credibility and standing with those around you. That increase is not designed to make you look cleverer or special, but to make you more influential.

The way you carry out your management role, even when you are not overtly trying to influence people, is in itself incredibly influential. We often have to tell participants on our management courses that, even if *they* consider themselves to be mere junior or middle managers, unable to make the big stuff happen, their management practice will be evaluated carefully by those around them. In fact, most junior managers are far more influential than they think they are, principally because, as far as their staff are concerned, their words and actions reflect the management regime of the whole organisation. In fact, just the mood, the emotional state, of the leader is highly influential and has been linked to staff retention and the degree of co-operation in the workforce.[1] Reviewing studies on this subject, Goleman suggests that even when they are not talking, the leader is watched more carefully than anyone else in the group. He concludes that 'the leader sets the emotional standard'.[1]

So it's clear that the way the manager behaves is important. It can certainly make the difference between a member of staff having a good and productive or a horrible day at work. If that is not being influential, we don't know what is!

INFLUENCING WITHOUT THINKING

Dov Frohman, founder of Intel Israel, writes:

> It took me years to realize just how powerful an impact my actions could have on employees … Once, for example, I chewed out a subordinate at a team meeting for some error (I forget

what). At the next meeting of the group, the individual didn't show up. I asked a colleague where the missing manager was – only to be informed that he had been so upset at my criticism that he had become ill!

Another time, lost in thought, I passed a colleague in the hallway without saying hello. It was only later that I learned that my silence had caused him considerable anxiety. Had he done something wrong? Was he no longer on my good side? My non-response, which was completely inadvertent, made him genuinely worried that he had done something to damage his standing in the organization.[2]

In this chapter we focus on two aspects of behaviour: the way you manage your own time and the way you cope when stressed. Both of these send powerful messages to your staff, peers and bosses. They can make the difference between you being a positive, successful influencer or merely a safe, but irrelevant, part of the management regime or even a loose cannon, influential but not in positive ways. Which do you want to be?

TIME MANAGEMENT

In general, we are better at managing our money than we are at managing our time. We get reminders (bank statements) of where our money has gone, some of us have computer software programs that help sort out budgets, and a few even make cost–benefit calculations in our heads before we go out and buy something desirable but not essential! Indeed, some of us delay or avoid making a purchase because, at the time, we do not have the money or we need those resources for something more urgent/important.

When it comes to our time, which is just as precious as, and even more limited than, our money, we pay almost no attention to how it is used, The mental energy that we do commit to the topic tends to be used moaning about where the time has gone. To a certain extent, money can be replaced, but time can never be repaid. Once today has gone, there is no way of getting it back so we need to be as sure as we can be that time will spent be on the right things and worth the effort.

One way to do this is to start treating your time as money. For example, someone earning £25,000 per year has a cost per hour of £13.00 (based on a 37-hour week). If you take off time for annual leave, the figure rises to more than £14.50 per hour or £116.00 per active day.

Over a year, therefore, huge amounts of money/time are committed to the jobs you do, and starting to treat our time as a precious asset is a prerequisite for using it effectively. There are two sets of demands on your time – the ones you make and the ones others make! This section offers advice on the first of these.

Your demands on your own time

Most of us, if we think about managing our time, start by looking at our interruptions, the things that others do to us that get in our way. Therein lies the problem. If we keep thinking that we are OK but everyone else needs to change, we will stay inefficient but without ever knowing why. Remember 'the enemy is out there' obstacle to learning we covered in Chapter 1? As we discovered in Chapters 2 and 3 on personality and culture, if you want someone to change their behaviour towards you, you have to make the first move, so let us concentrate on your own contribution to time pressures.

In no particular order, the common self-inflicted wounds are as follows.

➤ Messy desk.
➤ Lack of clear goals (for the whole job or for a specific time period – week, day, morning, etc.).
➤ No review of how the time is being spent at present.
➤ The carrier bag/briefcase of papers that accompanies you home at night.
➤ Double handling of paper (including electronic paper such as emails).
➤ Putting yourself at the mercy of the computer.
➤ Lack of a good filing/bring-forward system.
➤ No explicit purpose behind phone calls.
➤ Losing control of the diary (if you have one).
➤ Running or attending meetings with low value and outcomes.
➤ Not understanding when during the day you are at your most effective/ energetic/focused.

We do not expect that you will recognise all of these, but most managers who see they have a problem accept that at least a few are relevant to them. Here are some hints for addressing the ones that are on your own personal radar.

Messy desk

This is a sensitive one to start with because we know several people who have messy desks and who can put their hand on anything they need within seconds. However, they are in the minority. An untidy desk has been found to lose between two and five hours per week of productive time (depending on the type of job) finding stuff, redoing stuff, preparing material too quickly or damaging material whilst moving it around looking for other stuff. Everyone has periods where their paper mounts up but five minutes of tidying and sorting will pay dividends. Of course, your job may be less desk based than others and you might think this section is of less relevance to you. Beware that thought. If you spend the vast majority of your time in clinical areas and return to that desk infrequently, it is even more important that these brief visits are spent being productive, not wading through piles of unopened or opened and then disregarded mail, messages left days ago by well-meaning colleagues, and a pending tray bursting at the seams.

The material on any desk will fall into three broad categories.

➤ There for a reason.
➤ There in case.
➤ There for want of somewhere else to put or send it!

The first category of material should be on the desk when being worked on and in a known and organised storage system when not. (More on filing and bring-forward systems later.)

The second category should be off the desk, full stop. Otherwise it simply gets in the way of, or even hides, the important material and increases the chances of that important or urgent stuff being ignored until it is too late.

The third category should either not have come to you or, having served its purpose, should go somewhere else. That might be the bin, a bookcase or a work colleague (if it is likely to be of value to them).

Find a moment in the next few days, and start by marking what is on your desk using those three categories. Don't try to fix everything at once – you don't have the time and you probably don't have the willpower at this stage – but at least do something about the first category material, and have a quick look through the second category stuff to make sure nothing urgent has been buried.

SPINNING YOUR WHEELS OR DRIVING FORWARD?

In a *Harvard Business Review* article entitled 'Beware the busy manager', Bruch and Ghoshal[3] claim that only:

> … 10% of managers are purposeful – that is both highly energetic and highly focused. They use their time effectively by carefully choosing goals and then taking deliberate actions to reach them. Managers that fall into the other groups, by contrast, are usually just spinning their wheels; some procrastinate, others feel no emotional connection to their work, and still others are easily distracted from the task at hand. Although they look busy, they lack either the focus or the energy required for making any sort of meaningful change.

Clear goals

Many of us do not set clear goals, either for our lives or for our jobs. We may have objectives and targets, but these are rarely translated into what that means for our physical work programme today, or this week, or this month. The key here is to be realistic, bearing in mind this work on goal setting is for your eyes only! Whether you write the goals down or not is up to you but it can help if you start the week, or finish the week before with a few minutes of thinking about what you are trying to achieve over the next few days. If your work tends to come to you then this task will be a fairly modest one. If your work is largely self-generated, it becomes more important to map out your priorities and then act to protect time to achieve these. Without these regular times for reflection and planning, we end up in a dangerous loop whereby our lack of reflection leads to frantic but unfocused activity leading to lack of real progress which leads to increased busyness which, to complete the loop, leads to lack of reflection. If you are trapped in this loop, you need take action now!

Having clear goals is positive time management. Several of the hints in this section are concerned with avoiding or minimising the things that waste time, but the effect of clarity of purpose is that important activities will force out unimportant ones. Without a clear sense of what you are really trying to achieve in your job, you will find it impossible to know what to do first or what to say no to. This will result in lots of activity but little in the way of progress. In our coaching work, we find that most managers have difficulty controlling their workload. We ask them to think hard and identify the three or four things that they really want to accomplish in the next six months or year. These might be about building their team, improving their relationship with their boss, getting a particular project off the ground or achieving a new level of service. In defining these goals, they make it easier for themselves to choose between the many competing demands on their time.

One way to reality check the value and implications of a goal is to ask the following questions.

➤ Why do I think it is my goal/objective/priority and not someone else's?
➤ What would happen if I didn't do it?
➤ How long might it take (or) how much time does it deserve this week?
➤ What or whose help do I need to make progress, and are they likely to be available this week?

You may think of other more helpful questions, but even if this is an uncomfortable process for you, try to spend a few minutes sorting out your priorities.

Using a time log

Those of a self-disciplined and organised personality will take to this one much easier than you spontaneous and creative types, but it can be a real eye opener to log your use of time over a set period and then review what you actually spend your time doing. There is no one right way to do this. Some people design a simple form divided into periods of the day (normally 15 or 30 minutes) and write in what they were doing during that time, with whom, for what purpose and with what outcome.

Others simply jot the information in their diaries as they go along. It needs a bit of stamina but a log taken over a fortnight will normally be sufficient to give you quality data. Please don't keep doing it forever! Once you have the information you will see the following.

➤ How much of your time is self-determined and how much is taken by others' demands.

➤ The types of people who take most of your time. Many people find the 80/20 principle at work here – 80% of your interruptions are caused by 20% of the people, or 20% of your work tasks take up 80% of your time.

➤ Where you tend to drift or lose focus (this can help you establish productive times of the day or week (see later).

➤ Where you keep returning to the same task (which may tell you something about when it might be best to allocate a set time and finish a task). Studies have shown that an interrupted task can take up to 50% longer to complete than if it had been given adequate, protected time at the start.

➤ You will also see that some activities are more urgent than important, whereas others are more important than urgent. Delegate the unimportant, tackle the urgent now, and protect time for the important (see advice on diary management later).

Carrier bag/briefcase

Are you one of those people who put stuff in a bag or case at the end of each day, take it home and then bring it back the following day untouched. Why is that? Is it a status symbol, an expression of importance, a comfort blanket, or merely the result of too much to do during the day? Whatever the cause, the lack of attention overnight certainly doesn't solve the problem and can simply add to the guilt.

The medicine here is strong. If you are not going to work on it at home (and why should you unless it is a personal choice?), leave it at work. Use our other techniques to review why it is in the case in the first place but don't just leave stuff in the case to build up its own 'frequent flyer' points.

Handling each piece of paper/email just once

This sounds impossible or impracticable and in reality you will probably handle important stuff many times as you work on it. What this is saying is that if you pick up a piece of paper or read an email, do something with it there and then. The action could be a reply, a call, a deleting or throwing away, filing, setting to one side for full attention at a scheduled time, but please do not simply put it on a pile and then have to pick it up several times again just to work out what to do with it. Double and triple handling of paper and emails is a major time waster, and a contributor to the messy desk syndrome.

Control the computer!

Some software features designed to be helpful can actually get in our way! Email systems beep at you when an email arrives, almost demanding that you stop doing what you were doing to look at it. Having been interrupted, you read the message before either doing something temporary about it or going back to what you were doing before, thus adding to the double handling of paper mentioned above. It's the equivalent of your postman or woman ringing you at work to say that they have delivered a letter and would you return home to open it, and by the way they will be back later in the day with more letters! Switch the speakers off and read emails in batches at times that suit the rest of your day.

Email housekeeping is a dull but vital part of your time management arsenal. We predict that most of you have an email inbox with dozens of opened emails still in them. That is the equivalent of having opened and read 30 letters and then putting them all down in a pile 'until later'. Once read, every email should find a new home and Microsoft Outlook (or Apple's equivalent, Entourage) gives you lots of options. You can move them to a tasks list (a sort of electronic to-do list), delete them or archive them, forward them to someone else and then move them to a new folder marked for that person. You can even set up rules so that emails from particular people or about particular subjects can go to specific folders. This way the important topics or messages from key people will never get lost in a cluttered inbox. The gold standard here is that once an email has been read, it leaves the inbox. If you don't currently do this, then it will be a slog at the start but once done, it becomes natural and so helpful.

Filing and bring-forward systems

For most people, filing is a necessary evil and something to find others to do for you. A good filing system should be invisible – it just does the job and you do yours. A bad or non-existent filing system can seriously compromise your efficiency as you search for lost files, redo work unnecessarily, look unprofessional and raise your stress levels. The exact design of a system depends on the work you do and we cannot give you a 'one size fits all' template. But we do want to raise its importance with you and suggest that, if your current system does not do the job you want it to do, at least get together and make some changes. Find someone in your team who has an organised and detailed mind and get their advice.

Bring-forward (BF) systems are easier to implement individually, and can transform both your desk and your sense of being in control of your work. As the name suggests, it is a system that brings material back to you, at a time that suits both you and the task at hand. Typically a BF system consists of a number of hanging files, either in your desk drawer or filing cabinet. Some people have four, one for each week in a month, labelled 1–7, 8–14, 15–22, 23–31, whilst others with more precise schedules have one file for each day. Once a piece of paper comes in, it is either dealt with once straight away or marked with the date you want it back on your desk, and then placed in the appropriate folder. Each day, simply have a quick look in that folder and bring out what you need.

This approach prevents papers sitting on the desk, where they could get lost, hidden or damaged, and avoids the need to put them in a larger filing system where they may take more work to retrieve. Whether you are single-handed or part of a larger team, a bring-forward system can seriously improve confidence in your paper storage.

Phone calls

If you ring someone about a work issue, it is a good idea to introduce the purpose explicitly at the beginning. 'Hi Joe, do you have five minutes? Good, I have two things I need from you. The first is ...' This looks a little artificial out of context but there are two important ingredients. First, you establish that there is enough time in the call to complete the business. All too often you start a conversation only for the other person to have to go and so the call is repeated later and the original time is wasted. Second, you provide boundaries for the call – both you and the recipient know exactly why the call has been made and both are more likely to commit to achieving that purpose.

Diary management

Most of us, if we have a diary, would have to admit that it acts principally as a record and reminder of other people's demands on our time. We may have some of our priorities in there but they are likely to be a very small minority. Because of this, we get asked to do things or go to meetings by bosses and colleagues and, if the diary is 'free', we say yes and there goes another slice of the day. Remember the time was never free; it was simply not allocated against a piece of work or person at that time. But what about your work, your priorities and your needs? For many of you, regular appointments will be a major feature of your diary but if you have work to do outside those set times, when is it going to get done? Never, if the 'free' time keeps being offered to everyone else.

The simplest way of getting some balance in your diary is to book meetings with yourself. It's deceptively simple but unless you commit time to get your important stuff done, and demonstrate that in your diary, it will be too easy to put that work in the carrier bag and take it home. Balance is critical here. If you go overboard and fill every available slot with your work, you will never be available for social and work-related contact with colleagues, but if you do nothing, other demands will invade and take over. Start by booking an hour a week and protecting it 'to the death', even if you don't know exactly how it will be used. You will find that issues emerge and you can always release the time later if you wish. Just make sure you are the one making that choice.

Meetings: yes or no?

One of us knew a colleague whose mantra on meetings he was invited to was: 'no agenda – no thanks'. This does not mean he needed a formal agenda every time; what he wanted to know was why the meeting was being held, with what intended outcome and what contribution he was expected to make. The absence of answers would normally lead to him either declining or asking some straight questions before saying yes. The constraints of organisational life (particularly the Apollo culture we described in Chapter 3) can make this somewhat defiant approach difficult to do every time, but the more hawkish you are, the more meetings you can avoid and so use the time for other things. This also applies to meetings you call and organise. If you cannot see a clear purpose and potential beneficial outcome, you are risking a waste of your own time and that of others.

There are many other hints and tips on meetings management and these are contained in our first book *Essential Skills for Managing in Healthcare*, but the process starts with a commitment to only hold, or go to, meetings that you are confident will add value.

When are you most productive?

For some people this will seem a somewhat flaky theory, but others will readily accept that there are specific times of the day when they feel more productive, creative, focused or just plain calm. Most of us cannot use this self-awareness to simply dictate to our employers when we will turn up to work or get busy, but it can help to sort out the best time of day to do those tasks that are not themselves time bound. If you know that later afternoon is when you get a burst of energy and discipline, then you might allocate that time to correspondence, emails, reports, etc. Others find that early morning is thinking time and so they plan to get to their workplace 30 minutes before everyone else, not to push paper around but just get their head around personnel issues, difficult clients, etc.

Your time log may give you clues as to when that time is for you, or you may just have always known it. It terms of time management, the trick is to put that knowledge to work and protect those parts of your diary for the tasks that have the greatest pay-off for you.

STRESS MANAGEMENT

Next in our look at how to influence others by the way you manage yourself, we turn to how you cope with stress. For this we need to return to your self-assessment from Chapter 2.

If you remember, we looked at how the MBTI can be used to reveal your preferences for orientation, information gathering, decision making and lifestyle. If you completed the self-assessment, you will have arrived at an MBTI type, composed of four letters. We both have the type INFP (introverted, intuitive, feeling and perceiving) although yours is likely to be different.

The MBTI provides useful insights into the sorts of things that stress us, how we behave under stress and what we might do to minimise stress.

Causes of stress

You need firstly to be aware of what stresses you. A landmark UK study[4] into occupational stress found that, overall, the workplace characteristics most commonly associated with stress were as follows.

➤ Working long hours
➤ High exposure to noise
➤ Having to work fast
➤ High skill level required
➤ Taking the initiative
➤ Not being given enough information
➤ Having to combine different things
➤ High workload
➤ Responsibility
➤ Frequent interruptions
➤ Overtime
➤ Being treated unfairly
➤ No respect from others
➤ Inadequate support

However, what stresses one person may not stress another, and things that cause anxiety in one person may be energising for others. What constitutes 'frequent interruptions' may vary dramatically between different people. The characteristics associated with the various MBTI preferences suggest the following.

➤ Extraverts are more likely to experience stress if they are consistently or systematically denied opportunities to talk things through, be in company or have variety in their daily lives.
➤ Introverts are more likely to be stressed by seemingly endless external stimulus, prolonged social interaction without a break or having to constantly give out without respite.
➤ Sensing types tend to be stressed by others' inability or unwillingness to respect the evidence or by a requirement to make permanent decisions based on little or no evidence.

➤ Intuitives, as we might expect, are made anxious by being held back from focusing on the big picture and future possibilities, and may find having to wade through what seems to them impenetrable statistics not only boring but irritating and stressful.

➤ Thinking types may be stressed about decisions that have little objective logic or reason about them, or which to them appear to be made 'on the hoof' rather than through a rational process.

➤ In contrast, Feeling types may experience mild stress when feeling forced to consider only hard logic and impersonal judgements in their decision making, or when their wish to factor in people issues is derided by colleagues.

➤ Judging types may be uncomfortable with loose, unplanned arrangements that appear to leave everything to the last minute as, for them, this equates to high risk and implies a lack of professionalism.

➤ Finally, Perceiving types could experience stress when forced into step-by-step planning and early action, as this not only removes the fun for them but is likely to leave them feeling as if they are merely complying rather than truly engaging with the task.

Managing stress

One key to managing these situations is to plan ahead, however challenging that may be for you Perceiving types. Of course, you cannot predict every stressful situation – sometimes it is the suddenness that produces the stress. However, look at the day or week in front of you and try to spot where the stresses might build up. For example, is there a meeting coming up with someone who presses all the wrong buttons with you? Will you be put under pressure to justify a proposal to your boss, and how did you react the last time they started to undermine your arguments? Once you can see when and where the stresses might come from, then you can factor in some 'me time', which allows you to reset the balance. Look for activities and pastimes that work with the grain of your natural preferences and protect even just a few minutes within the forthcoming period for those experiences. Given that we can cope quite well with being outside our preferences, you may not need long to reset your internal scales.

Another key is to delegate wisely or exchange the activities that stress you. Remember, different people find different things stressful and the task that you dread may be easier or even pleasurable for someone else in your team. The painstaking statistical analysis that drives you to distraction might be the sort of task that a colleague with an eye for detail and a preference for order and logic would relish. In return, you could help them with the strategic report that they are struggling with. We would remind you, though, that we said 'delegate wisely'. We might add 'sensitively'. We don't advise or condone simply dumping on other people the bits of your job that you don't like. That is merely moving stress around the organisation. But careful consideration and some thoughtful discussion with colleagues are likely to expose opportunities for redistributing tasks in a way that is more suited to the personalities involved. One word of warning: while too many activities that go against the grain of who you are is a recipe for unhealthy stress, we all need some discomfort and challenge in order to keep learning and growing.

Finally, if having tried these approaches, your job is still too stressful, you might well need a change of role. This could be as simple as redesigning your role within your current organisation or as drastic as a change of career. Only you can decide if this is necessary but if you are in a role that is continually making you anxious and worried, you owe it yourself and to those close to you to take action. Stress can have a whole range of undesirable consequences including sleeping difficulties, depression or even heart disease,[5] quite apart from the impact it may have on your friends and family.

Behaviour under stress: losing our balance

Even with good planning and a sensible work–life balance, there will be times when we experience stress. It could be an unexpected need to work late, a complaint that seems unjustified but which leads to heavy criticism or perhaps conflict with a fellow worker. At such times we may begin to lose our cool or perspective.

According to MBTI theory, each of us has a preferred mental process, called the dominant function. It's the part of our personality type that we most trust and rely on to get us through life and consequently it is very close to the core of who we are. Normally, this dominant function is balanced and complemented by the other parts of our personality but under stress, when things seem to be getting out of control, we may begin to overuse this favourite part of ourselves to regain a sense of control and order. Unfortunately, our over-reliance on one aspect of our personality leads us to become unbalanced. It is sometimes called the 'exaggerated state'[6] because one aspect of our personality starts to dominate and our behaviour may become a little like a caricature of how we are at our best.

Take us as an example. We are both INFP and the dominant function of an INFP is Feeling which, because we are Introverts, is used on the inside. Under stress, if our Introverted Feeling begins to take control, our normal concern for people turns into a feeling that we alone can help them and that we alone are carrying the world's problems. Our normal self-reliance and independence become isolation. We may also become a little 'preachy' as we see our personal values and ideals as all-important. Also, our normal sensitivity becomes a tendency to take everything personally.

Use the table below, based on work by Nancy Barger and Linda Kirby,[7] to see what being out of balance might look like for your type.

Type	Dominant function	Possible behaviour under stress
ENFP, ENTP	Extraverted Intuition	Big picture thinking becomes a fixation with links or patterns Energy and drive become frenetic activity Ability to be flexible and see possibilities becomes indecision or sudden changes of direction
ISTJ, ISFJ	Introverted Sensing	Carefully thinking things through becomes an inability to act Concern for facts becomes obsession with detail Confidence in own judgement becomes inflexibility Selective communication becomes no communication
INTJ, INFJ	Introverted Intuition	Ability to see links and patterns in data becomes overcomplexity Independence becomes inability to ask for help Visionary thinking becomes detached from reality
ESTP, ESFP	Extraverted Sensing	Straightforwardness becomes bluntness Concern for detail becomes pedantic Action orientation becomes acting without thinking
ESFJ, ENFJ	Extraverted Feeling	Concern for people becomes intrusive Seeking harmony becomes peace which avoids underlying issues Concern for others becomes overburdened with worry
ISTP, INTP	Introverted Thinking	Concern for logic becomes insistence that their logic is best Objectivity becomes detachment Depth of thought becomes lost in thought
ISFP, INFP	Introverted Feeling	Independent stance becomes separation from others Sensitivity becomes oversensitivity Idealism becomes belief that their ideals are the only ones
ESTJ, ENTJ	Extraverted Thinking	Objectivity becomes critical detachment Clarity becomes oversimplification Concern for logic becomes insistence on logic Objective analysis becomes harsh criticism

Knowing how we might act under stress helps us to recognise the behaviours and, hopefully, moderate them. We may also gain insight into why others respond to our out-of-balance selves in the way they do.

If you become aware that you, or someone else, is losing balance, it is a good idea to press the pause button and allow some time for balance to be restored. If you are in a meeting, suggest a coffee break or comfort break. If you can, try to go for a quick walk or shift your focus to another task.

In the grip

If the stressful circumstances worsen and there is no respite, a more extreme reaction may occur. MBTI practitioners call this being 'in the grip' because instead of the strongest, most preferred part of our personality taking control, severe stress results in the parts of us we least understand and least identify with erupting with unpleasant or upsetting consequences. We are then *in the grip* of ways of thinking that are unskilled and which have a negative cast. In the grip, we may act in ways that seem very out of character even to people who know us well. This is reflected in commonly heard phrases like:

➤ I don't know what came over me
➤ Someone else just took over
➤ She just flipped.

People who are normally objective and decisive can display sudden bursts of emotion. Practical, grounded types may start to have negative flights of imagination where they see everything going wrong. Big picture types might become obsessive about facts and details and people who are normally caring and people focused may suddenly become highly critical and judgemental. While they are in the grip, each person feels justified in their thinking, even if to those around them the behaviour seems extreme or inexplicable. Because of this, reasoning with someone in the grip will not work. It may just make things worse. The best course of action, as we discussed above, is to take time out. If you recognise the signs of severe stress, you need to take some time well away from the circumstances that stress you. When you can, begin to reflect on what happened or what is happening and maybe talk this through with someone to see what can be learned. If you think you may have upset or offended someone, don't beat yourself up but go and put things right with them.

In the grip episodes are less often encountered than the out-of-balance behaviour we explored earlier in the chapter and for that reason we will not spend much time on the subject. For a fuller explanation of being in the grip and what you can do about it, we recommend Naomi Quenk's excellent book *Was That Really Me?*.

Setting an example

So far, we have looked at you and your own coping mechanisms for stress. However, this section is also about the example you set to others. Things you can do to support your staff include the following.

➤ Making stress discussible. This can normalise the situation and give people permission to be larger than life sometimes without feeling condemned.
➤ Support your staff in identifying the things that stress them and work with them to either minimise those aspects of the job or provide support mechanisms for when they cannot be avoided.

➤ Build in review sessions at regular intervals during the life of a project or after particularly stressful periods for your team. Use them to revisit not only the successes and challenges of the work but also the ways in which individuals coped. It is vital that this activity is carried out in the spirit of openness and learning, not judgement and defensiveness. It may lead to people being assigned different roles next time, roles that play to their strengths, and it will almost certainly lead to greater peer support through the difficult times.

As with most acts of leadership, you must demonstrate the behaviours that you wish to see in others, so start by asking the team to review your own performance. If you do not, your credibility will suffer and your ability to influence others in future will be diminished.

Conclusion

As we conclude this section on stress, please note these three things.

➤ A degree of stress is both normal and necessary. Unless we experience some tension or frustration with situations, we are unlikely to have either the motivation to change things or the adrenalin to do well.

➤ Admitting to stress must never be used to determine a person's value or future opportunities to succeed. As soon as the trust necessary to encourage disclosure is lost, the stresses will not go away, but will go underground where they are far more damaging to the work of your team and the health of the individual.

➤ A mature approach to stress management can be a powerful team-building tool. Teams that are open and genuinely supportive tend to be more successful than those fuelled by suspicion and disloyalty. This does not mean that all good teams are warm and fluffy environments where tension is absent. Quite the opposite – many teams need the spark of creative tension for new ideas to emerge and for the status quo to be challenged. What sets these teams apart is that they know when things are getting superheated and they help each other to cope. Which sort of team would you like to lead or be part of?

In summary, you must not underestimate the degree of influence you can wield just by the way you behave and the way you cope with the unexpected. Please do not be fooled by your position on the organisation chart or by the number of staff in your team. Most of us make our real judgements about someone by the way they behave, even if we sometimes have to work professionally with those we do not regard particularly highly.

In our last book we suggested that the mark of a good manager is someone of whom others will say 'I can do business with that person'. The word 'person' is critical here. You may disagree strongly with the proposal or argument put forward by that other person. Indeed, they may vehemently oppose your point of view. However, as long as your own integrity is intact, you will continue to be influential. Indeed, the way you deal with those arguments will heavily influence the way that other person relates to you next time.

Not all influence comes from the power of your evidence or the devastating logic of the case you are putting forward. If it did, we could dispense with face-to-face discussions and simply commit all proposals to computer-driven analysis. Outside the work environment as well as inside, we deal with people and we tend to trust and listen to those who, without being overbearing or egotistical, have good self-management skills and just seem to be 'on top of things'.

If you can improve your time management and your handling of stressful situations, you will send a powerful and reassuring message to those around you that you too are 'on top of things' and are a person whom others can do business with.

FURTHER READING

➤ For more on managing stress, try *Work Types* by Jean Kummerow, Nancy Barger and Linda Kirby, published by Business Plus.

➤ For more on being 'in the grip', try *Was That Really Me?* by Naomi Quenk, published by Davies-Black.

REFERENCES

1 Goleman D. *The New Leaders*. London: Sphere; 2002.
2 Frohman D. *Leadership the Hard Way*. San Francisco: Jossey-Bass; 2008. pp.80–1.
3 Bruch H, Ghoshal S. Beware the busy manager. *Harvard Bus Rev*. 2002; **February**: 62–9.
4 Health and Safety Executive. *The Scale of Occupational Stress: The Bristol Stress and Health at Work Study*. 2000. www.hse.gov.uk/research/crr_pdf/2000/crr00265.pdf
5 Institute of Work, Health and Organisations. *Work Organisation and Stress*. www.who.int/occupational_health/publications/en/oehstress.pdf
6 Kummerow J, Barger N, Kirby L. *Work Types*. New York: Business Plus; 1997. p.208.
7 Barger N, Kirby L. *The Challenge of Change in Organizations*. Palo Alto: Davies-Black; 1995.

CHAPTER 7

Summary and next steps

In this chapter, we'll draw the threads together and suggest how you can continue your learning journey. We hope we've convinced you that being influential is not a competence to be achieved or a set of facts to be acquired. Instead, it is a process of becoming more open to learning about yourself and others, even when the learning challenges what you previously thought to be true. This is harder than mastering a technique, but much more worthwhile.

We also hope you will agree that influencing is much more than just selling. The good manager influences not just through words and not just at certain times. The good manager influences continually through example, bringing hope and wisdom through actions as well as words. And whether they are conscious of it or not, people respond to this integrity – this matching up of words and deeds – with trust, even if they may disagree with what you are trying to do. When they feel they are being 'sold' a managerial message or when someone appears to act inconsistently, such trust is impossible.

SO MUCH TO DO!

Confronted with lessons about culture, personality, learning, change, etc., etc., you may be wondering where to start and what to do. In this concluding chapter, we'll help you reflect on the book's main messages and suggest some next steps.

We are conscious that we're setting the bar high. We're asking you to embrace learning that will challenge not just your intellect but also your ideas of who you are and what you see as important. And while we don't see our goal as making people uncomfortable, we do see some discomfort and self-examination as integral to real learning. Perhaps the book has prompted a few wry smiles or 'aha' moments as you've seen why well-intentioned but mistaken influencing attempts failed to produce the desired result. We invite you to work on these areas and not leave improvement to chance.

We have set out these challenges not just to help you have a more successful career but because the way we deal with each other in organisations is important. People's happiness and motivation depend on our ability to influence with integrity rather than with the sole aim of winning. This becomes even more important in healthcare organisations when patient care can be undermined by poor morale and distrust.

For each person reading this book, different challenges and lessons will come to the fore. Depending on your history and circumstances, some of the book's messages will have much more relevance than others. As we review the chapters, note the themes and issues that made the most impact on you.

CHAPTER 1: LEARNING TO INFLUENCE

In this chapter we saw how learning that changes us – real learning – can be uncomfortable. This is because we may have to discard long-held assumptions about ourselves and other people. We discussed how people avoid or defend against this kind of learning by blaming others or taking action that is not sufficiently thought through or which does not address the real issue. We suggested some practical ways in which you can increase your ability to learn, such as keeping a learning journal or using active listening.

Main messages from Chapter 1

➤ Learning by experience is not guaranteed.
➤ We all, at times, resist learning. But this resistance may be unconscious and we will find reasons to justify our reluctance to change how we act.
➤ Active listening, team learning and keeping a learning journal can help us become better learners.

CHAPTER 2: LEARNING ABOUT YOURSELF

The main theme of this chapter is the importance of self-awareness and awareness of how others may differ from you in terms of personality and, therefore, how they prefer to be influenced. We offered the MBTI as a tool you can use to better understand yourself and how you come across.

Main messages from Chapter 2

➤ Management and influencing are primarily about people.
➤ Self-awareness is central to good management and wise managers actively seek out feedback.
➤ Appraisal and personality inventories such as the MBTI are good sources of feedback.

➤ When influencing, we need to take into account the fact that others think and make decisions in different ways.

CHAPTER 3: ORGANISATIONAL CULTURE

Here, we explored the ways in which organisations differ, not just in terms of size or function but also in terms of culture. Culture, although not written down and usually invisible to those who are in it, has a large bearing on what types of influencing approach will succeed. We used Harrison's model of culture as a way of identifying cultures frequently encountered in healthcare organisations and we suggested what approaches might work in each culture.

Main messages from Chapter 3

➤ We need to respect and take account of the culture of a team or individual when attempting to influence them, even if we don't particularly like it.
➤ Influencing approaches which work well in our 'home' culture may be entirely useless or even counterproductive in another setting.
➤ Find out what culture you are dealing with through research or questioning.

CHAPTER 4: INFLUENCING ORGANISATIONAL CHANGE

There is good evidence that simply telling people what to do is an ineffective way to bring about change in organisations. To successfully influence change, we need to remember that organisations are made up of people and that change is primarily a human, rather than technical, issue. Rather than using force or manipulation to get people to comply, the wise manager involves people in the change, giving them a voice and making use of their insight and creativity. We suggested new principles for change management that acknowledge the humanity of organisations.

Main messages from Chapter 4

➤ Organisational change cannot be controlled, only led or influenced. Command and control approaches are neither sustainable nor effective.
➤ Change needs to be treated as a process or a journey, not an event.
➤ If allowed to become constructively involved, staff are an asset in change rather than an obstacle.

CHAPTER 5: INFLUENCING IN FORMAL SETTINGS

Influencing sometimes has to be carried out in formal settings. Although the messages from other chapters still apply, the formal nature of the process demands a modified approach. This chapter offers guidance on how to prepare for and carry out formal influencing.

Main messages from Chapter 5

➤ Formality offers challenges but also provides opportunities for you to be seen as professional and trustworthy.

➤ Structure and process can help diffuse tension.

➤ As with other forms of influencing, doing some research and then matching your style to that of the other party(ies) will pay dividends.

➤ Work out 'what it is in it' for the other parties and pursue mutual benefit, not win/lose.

➤ Remember you will have to work with these people the next day, and the day after, so build a reputation for trustworthiness, not aggression.

CHAPTER 6: BEING A ROLE MODEL

This chapter argues that influencing is as much about how we act as what we say. The way we manage our time, handle ourselves under stress and control our workload sends strong messages to our colleagues about what is really important to us, regardless of what we might say. We offer some very practical advice on being a good role model and we return to the MBTI to help you understand how stress might affect your behaviour.

Main messages from Chapter 6

➤ The way we act is influential. Good managers are good role models.

➤ Time is a resource to be managed thoughtfully.

➤ It is possible to create a more productive work environment through managing emails and paper.

➤ We behave differently under stress. Understand the things that stress you and take action to minimise the negative effects.

DECIDING WHAT IS IMPORTANT FOR YOU NOW

This book offers insights into many areas and suggests many ways to be more influential. But you can't do them all at once. Having now summarised the book's main messages, the next section is designed to help you identify what areas might be most relevant to you.

Don't rush through the questions that follow. Take some time to think about them carefully. Minimise other distractions and devote some time to your development.

Step 1: areas for learning

Write down the areas where you would most like to see personal learning and change. This could be because the area interests you or because of your current work objectives or because of frustrations in your current role. It may be that you are just interested in personality issues and would like to be much more self-aware. Or it could be that your dealings with other professions or organisations have proved perplexing and you want to be able to navigate better through the difficult terrain of organisational culture. It might be that you are fed up with living with an over-flowing in-box and going home late every night and you'd like to learn to manage your time more effectively. Limit yourself to just three areas and, for each one, write in the table below the changes you'd like to see. For example, you might choose the area of being a role model in the way you manage your time, and the changes you'd like to see might include regularly leaving work before 6pm. Remember that the focus is on you, and that the changes you want to see all must start with you. Hopefully your boss and your colleagues will be supportive, but the impetus and initiative must come from you.

Learning area	Changes I'd like to see
e.g. learning to be a role model in how I manage my time	e.g. leaving work before 6pm most nights, having time for regular staff appraisals
1	
2	
3	

Step 2: possible development actions

For each of the three learning areas you chose in step 1, write down one or two things you could do to learn and develop and bring about the changes you want to see. You may find it helpful to return to the chapter that deals with the issue you are writing about, as each chapter contains suggestions for enhancing your learning or improving your performance. These suggestions include further reading, practical tips for time management, active listening and planning for formal influencing. Note down your potential development actions using the table below.

Learning area	Possible development actions
e.g. improve team learning	e.g. organise team time-out
1	
2	
3	

Step 3: next steps – committing to action

Depending on your personality, this may be the part you've been impatiently waiting for or the part you'd prefer to delay or avoid! Much as we accept that life cannot be planned in detail and that things will always happen to surprise us, we also believe that without firm intentions we will never achieve very much. So, whether you are a planner or the kind of person who likes to let life unfold, we think you'll find it helpful to decide what you are going to do next about your development as an influencer.

Re-read what you have written in steps 1 and 2 and then note down the next three things you will do to start turning your good intentions into action. For instance, if the development action you most want to carry out is to sort out your in-box, write down when you will set aside time to do this. If you want to have a team time-out, note when you will organise this and who you will ask to facilitate it. Or if you are interested in taking the MBTI questionnaire, write down the next step, which may be researching how you can do this. You get the idea. What we're asking you to do is to make a commitment to yourself. But don't be overambitious. Just start with three things you can do in the next few days and then move onto something else. Use the table overleaf to note down your commitments.

The development actions I will take	What I need to do next	When I will do this by
e.g. take full MBTI questionnaire	Contact training department	Friday
1		
2		
3		

OVER TO YOU!

Learning is part of being a good manager and a good professional. Certainly, you can never hope to be an effective influencer without staying open to learning, whatever its source. And while no one can do our learning for us, equally no one can stop us from learning and growing. Even the frustrations we encounter, people who appear to stand in the way and obstacles that appear to block our path are, in themselves, the raw materials we need for personal transformation. By choosing to reflect and take action, rather than blame or bemoan our lot, we turn these raw materials into valuable learning.

Do let us know how you get on. We'd love to hear your stories about the joys (and pains!) of developing your influencing abilities. If you'd like to email us, the address is andrew@developmentconsultancy.co.uk.

So, onwards to successful influencing!

Index